# KNOTS, LINES, AND LIFE

# KNOTS, LINES, AND LIFE

## A JOURNEY THAT TORE ME APART AND PUT ME BACK TOGETHER

ASHTON PIENAAR

Star of Bravo's *Below Deck*

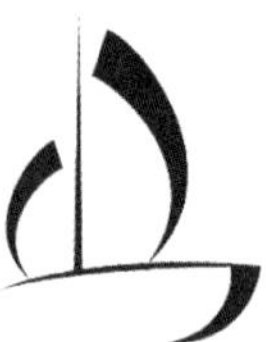

Ballast Books, LLC
www.ballastbooks.com



ISBN: 978-1-955026-60-4

Printed in Hong Kong

Published by Ballast Books
www.ballastbooks.com

For more information, bulk orders, appearances, or speaking requests,
please email: info@ballastbooks.com

# CONTENTS

"A ship in harbor is safe, but that is not what ships are built for."

John A. Shedd

"There is nothing more enticing, disenchanting, and enslaving than the life at sea."

Joseph Conrad

"Uncertainty is essential—and your path to freedom."

Deepak Chopra

# PROLOGUE

As our yacht left port in Puna'auia, Tahiti, with the sun warming my skin and a breeze carrying the rich smell of saltwater, I breathed in deep. *I can't believe this is my life,* I thought, feeling an increasingly familiar sense of awe. Working as a deckhand on a massive, beautiful yacht, traveling the world under clear skies with clean air and breathtaking views everywhere I turned, I felt overwhelmed with gratitude. Life hadn't always been this good.

Dressed in shorts and a polo shirt with boat shoes and a cap, I made my way to the aft deck, looking to help out after finishing my last task on the bow. Once we had successfully let the yacht loose from the dock and made our way out of the marina, our next high-pressure maneuver was releasing the tender[1] from the hip of the yacht to tow behind us.

By the time I got to the aft deck, the crew had already begun with the procedure, but I noticed the line that they'd let go from the midship, which let the front of the tender start drifting out and away from the yacht, had hooked around one of the fenders. So, I quickly hopped down onto the swim platform and unhooked the line, then followed it, intending to prevent it from catching on anything else. As I talked to my crewmate, cautioning her to be wary of the line, I took

1 A motorboat that accompanies a yacht, used for skiing and other activities as well as transporting guests to and from the yacht when they want to visit beaches and other ports along our journey.

one wrong step, thrusting me into a scenario more dangerous than any situation I'd yet encountered.

Something pulled at my foot, and when I looked down, I saw that the part of the tow line that had not yet paid out, which, moments before, had been lying harmlessly on the deck, was caught firmly around my ankle.

*OH, CRAP!*

I felt my body switch over to survival mode. A rush of adrenaline took over my thinking, as if I were Sherlock Holmes methodically planning out his next moves in slow motion. I, too, was assessing the situation at hand and calculating my next action. With one more second of tension left in the line I was holding between my hand and where it had caught my ankle, I gripped the line as tight as I could, looked at my crewmate next to me, and matter-of-factly said, "I'm going in."

As I fell, I turned my body so my back hit the water first. I was still holding tight to the line, hoping to use it to control what was about to happen next. Despite the predicament I found myself in, I couldn't let go. In a sense, it was my lifeline. If I hadn't held fast, I could've hit my head while being whipped wildly off the back of the boat by my ankle. Then, I would've been screwed because I'd have been tied up in the line, unconscious, guaranteed to be ripped apart by the line as it took full tension between the yacht and the tender. Put simply, I'd have been dead! So, I kept control. I held that bit of tension in my hand. My thought was, *If I can maintain control in this moment and just unloop this line from my ankle when I hit the water, I'll be able to swim off to the side, and I'll be fine.*

Seawater rushed into my nose, and panic filled my chest as I felt my body being pulled in different directions. I hadn't calculated for this before surrendering to my fate of being pulled off the deck. Not only was I being pulled forward, but I was being pulled down under the water too. I held my breath and dunked below the surface to try to unloop the line, but I quickly realized it wasn't going to be that simple. The line was clenched around my ankle in what felt like a vicelike grip.

See, there are two lines that go from each side of the yacht and then connect to a spectra line in the middle. My foot had actually gotten caught in the middle of this bridle where these lines all met and hooked up, creating an eye. That meant I was trying to unloop the line, thinking that it was just wrapped once around my ankle, but it had actually tightened from three separate points around my ankle. So, if I wanted to get out, I had to get my fingers between my skin and the lines and pull away in three different directions to open up that eye.

Unfortunately, I didn't realize how hopelessly bound I was, and my brain couldn't calculate additional solutions. My only idea had been to unloop the line. However, that wasn't happening, no matter how desperately I tried. *What am I going to do now?*

If you've ever done any type of water skiing, you know that when you first start being pulled behind the boat, you don't just pop up above the water. There's first a force that wants to naturally pull you down. Then, because you're on skis, you're able to push against that, lift the front of the skis, and get to the top and above the water. Of course, in this instance, I didn't have skis, yet I was being pulled forward as if I were being towed behind the boat. So, I was being dragged down behind the boat, and I had to fight to get my head above water to get some air.

I knew that if this line took tension, I was in big trouble. So, I took a deep breath and went under as a last-ditch attempt to try to freaking unloop this thing . . . but I just couldn't do it. In that moment, I was consumed by pure panic. It was paralyzing. My mind was rendered utterly frozen, so instead of trying something different, I just continued attempting what I'd already tried, thinking that I hadn't done it properly, but it was no use.

I still had some control of the line in my one hand, which allowed me to keep myself somewhat upright, controlling the way I was being dragged through the water. Otherwise, I would have been pulled feet first toward the boat, making it incredibly difficult to get my hands down to my ankle.

Before long, the tension started pulling, and it was too strong for me to hold the bend in my arm. As my arm snapped straight, I lost the little control I had. Suddenly, I was being pulled irresistibly by my ankle, and I could feel the force of the line tightening . . . tightening . . . tightening . . .

It all happened so quick. In this moment that felt like an eternity, I realized that this force was bigger than me. It was nothing like I felt in karate or rugby. Nobody had ever hit me that hard. Nothing had ever overwhelmed my body with such power. This was much mightier than my own strength or will.

The second the line started tightening with overpowering intensity, my foot started coming up out of the water because the line was fully taut. Now, there was no denying that I was facing something serious—deadly serious. I was in the unyielding grip of the spectral line, which was devastatingly sharp and strong enough to cut through human flesh like a knife. So, if the force strangling my ankle continued unimpeded, it would completely sever straight through my ankle.

As the struggle came to a climax, I essentially surrendered. *Okay, you lost this battle*, I admitted to myself. *You weren't able to get out of this line. Now, you are a victim to this situation. You've just got to grit your teeth and get through it.* The force was now getting past that point that I could tolerate it, and all I could do was release myself to my fate and accept that this was something I was going to have to endure.

Incredibly, in accepting that inescapable fact, I felt all fear leave me and, with it, all tension and resistance and will to fight. I felt peace. I didn't know exactly what would happen next, but I felt fairly certain that with these two massive forces pulling me in opposite directions, I was about to be torn apart.

In many ways, that was the story of my life.

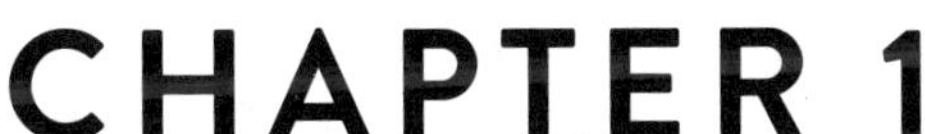

# CHAPTER 1

My life began as a surprise. My mom became pregnant with me at sixteen years old, and my father was seventeen. The subsequent chaos would shape me from the moment of conception—in some ways I would feel but not fully comprehend until decades later.

Before I was born, my parents decided to get married and attempt to go about raising me in the traditional fashion. Unfortunately, by the time I reached age five, their relationship wasn't working out, so they decided to divorce. I do not have pleasant memories of their time together. Mostly, I remember brutal fights, shouting and screaming, and the sound of items being smashed and shattered. That violence would follow me throughout my life like thunder echoing between mountains.

My father moved to the north of Johannesburg while my mother remained in the south, thirty-five minutes apart, setting the tone for my life as one of constantly being on the move. For the next several years, I mostly lived with my mom, traveling back and forth every other weekend to visit my father.

At the time, navigating two different homes just felt normal, although now I can see how all of this set a tone for me to expect that kind of unsettled disruption throughout my life. I became comfortable in chaos, yet I also sometimes felt compelled to seek it out—and, in more unfortunate circumstances, create it. But as a child, life felt relatively peaceful, despite the constant commute and uncertainty of what might happen next with my parents.

Even from that young age, however, I craved the bond of family. I felt close enough with my mother, who had lost much of her family over the years. My uncle and her younger brother, Wayne, passed away around the time I was two years old, and her father—my grandfather—passed away shortly after that when I was seven. For one reason or another, I never saw much of the rest of her side of the family other than her mom, my grandmother.

Both my parents were young and dealt with the same challenges most young people encounter. Through it all, they were both warm and loving and gave me everything I needed. I always felt loved and cared for. They were amazing parents while also managing the struggles of life. They were still figuring things out, finding their place in the world, doing the best they could. Of course, they weren't perfect—no one is—but they always ensured I had everything I needed and I felt like a priority. Looking back, I'm hugely appreciative that they were able to set their teenage years and early twenties aside, but they were fully devoted to me growing up. Although they were young, they both had decent jobs and did well for themselves and for our family. The only thing they ultimately struggled with was their relationship with each other.

Growing up with my dad, we always did active things. He had a Kawasaki super bike, and I would ride on the back of it with him. It was so fun! My dad was awesome—truly my hero. He always gave me a lot of responsibility as a little boy, allowing me to test certain boundaries and try things.

For example, he would let me feel the force of the kite that was pulling so I could understand how it worked. He also raced rubber ducks[2] designed to punch through waves and ramp over them, and I have great memories associated with that. In addition, I was never

2 Small, fast speedboats built on aerodynamic rubber pontoons.

allowed to touch the pellet gun on my own, but my dad let me try it with him and learn how to use it safely.

I did always feel like my dad was living on the edge—he was always doing something exciting and perhaps even daring and dangerous to an extent. I have amazing memories with him, playing catch, experiencing new things, and just living life to the fullest.

Soon enough, my dad met another woman and fell in love again. I could tell he was happy with this new woman, which made me happy too. Then, when I was around eight years old, my dad and his fiancée had a son, giving me a new baby half-brother. In some ways, being with them gave me a sense of family. I loved visiting them and longed to be with them more than just on the weekends.

One of my worst memories from my childhood occurred one weekend when my parents were having a dispute over child support. I was with my mom at a family friend's home three houses up to the street perpendicular to the one we lived on. From where I was standing looking out their living room window, I could see my dad pull up and wait for me. When I didn't come out, my dad contacted my mom, but she did not answer his calls or let him know that we would not be there. I was distraught, crying uncontrollably at the fact that she would not let me go with him. Seeing his confusion, knowing that he was there for me, was torture for me. To this day, that moment saddens me!

Perhaps the closest sense of family I experienced growing up came in the form of my friend Jacques, whom I attended elementary school with, as well as his sisters and their parents, Uncle Kosie[3] and Aunt Josi. And perhaps it was because I felt that Jacques was the brother I just never had growing up and his sisters felt like my sisters. In many instances, Uncle Kosie and Aunt Josi treated me just like their own child. Even when Jacques and I needed disciplining, I would get the same punishment! In many ways, I guess I could just feel that this was what a functional family was meant to be.

3 In South African culture, even if they are not your uncle by family, you call your elders "Uncle" and "Auntie" as a sign of respect.

Their home had lots of room and even a pool in the backyard, so we'd often go swimming there while they'd braai. Other times, we'd ride scooters around the neighborhood and go to the nearby mall to see a movie. On Sundays, when realtors were hosting open houses in the neighborhood, we would scooter around, find the fanciest houses, and pretend to be the rich children of parents who were on their way to see the home. Some weekends, Jacques's family would even take me with them to their house on Vygeboom Dam, where we would go skiing and wakeboarding, play cricket and volleyball, and drive quads around the area.

They treated me with love and warmth, and to me, they felt like what a family should feel like. For all of the unknowns in life, your family should be the people who always have your back.

As I mentioned, I began to feel that way about my dad and his fiancée too—enough that, by age twelve, I knew that I wanted to live with them. My parents agreed to that new arrangement, so I moved into my dad's place for good. Of course, this was a very difficult conversation for me to have with my mom as I knew that it would hurt her. That was a huge decision I had to make in the first years of being a teenager, but I believe it worked out well, and it didn't change how much I loved both my mom and my dad.

Even after that, I adored Jacques's family so much that when I would return to the south of JoBurg to stay with my mom, I'd end up spending three-quarters of my time at Jacques's house. My mom hated that and complained often, but Jacques was my best friend!

By this point, I had another little brother, and nothing brought me more joy than being Tristan's older brother. At the same time, as anyone with younger siblings can understand, things simply changed once I was no longer the only kid in the house. This was one of life's biggest lessons for me at this period of my life—learning that the world does not only revolve around me. In many ways, my fairytale life with my dad was not completely the same, as his time with me was divided. That didn't take away from how much I loved my brother, of course, but it certainly created a new dynamic in the household.

So, all in all, through the first couple of years living with my dad, I felt good and secure—everything I'd always wanted in a family. It wasn't perfect, but I was happy. Around the time I started high school, however, things began to change, and once again, my life became chaos.

# CHAPTER 2

On weekends when I was with my mom, my dad would often disappear for a while. He would never miss out on a weekend with me, but sometimes, he would show up at home an hour or two after I arrived after my weekend away. Since I would be just coming back from my mom's at that point, I wouldn't necessarily know what had happened. I'd just sense that there was some issue without recognizing exactly what the problem was. Basically, I would pick up on parts of arguments between my dad and his fiancée. From those little bits, I would piece together that he hadn't been there the whole weekend or had come home super late. There was tension between the two of them that was impossible to miss.

As this happened more frequently, so did fights between my dad and his fiancée, which would often escalate into terrifying screaming matches that involved the smashing and breaking of doors and other things. Of course, this was reminiscent of the situations with him and my mother. Later in life, I would make some discoveries about my father that would help explain this behavior, but as a teenager, all I knew was that my family was falling apart.

In time, my dad and his fiancée separated, and just like that, at fifteen years old, I felt like I'd lost a stepmother and a brother. The following years were characterized by more disruption as my dad dated new girlfriends. We would move in with them, they would break up, and we'd move out again.

Even though these girlfriends were all nice and loving to me, I could never get invested in the situation because I never knew what was coming next. After all, my dad was dating and looking for the right person for him, and most of these girlfriends didn't end up being the right partner. However, he didn't stop trying. I was going through all this with my dad, and I had to accept it for what it was because I never knew how long a relationship would last. Perhaps this newest girlfriend would be "the one," and it would be permanent, but it could also go the other way.

Later on, it became apparent that this had a significant effect on many of my own behaviors and relationships as I got older. However, these experiences also helped me become a strong-willed, hard-working, extremely motivated person as well. Rather than buckling under the pressure, I developed a simple, straightforward approach to the challenges of chaos. When turmoil took hold, I put my mind on two questions: *How can I deal with this? What are my solutions?* Now, having learned about the spiritual laws of success, I can see that this was really me asking myself one question: *What is the security I can find in this unknown?*

This would later become my mantra. However, at this stage of my life, I am not sure where my hunger for success came from. I believe it may have had something to do with sports, always wanting to push myself harder and perform better. Maybe it was my escape or way of coping with my unstable environment. It was the one thing I actually did have control over. There was always just this fire in me to be better and do better. It was like I was always just working toward creating a better future for myself. I was always super grateful for my parents and the things I would go through with them, but instead of the hard times getting me down, I turned them into learning opportunities.

Since I lacked a sense of harmony and calm in my home life, I came to find stability and security in accomplishment. The gym became a sanctuary for me, and sports such as cricket and rugby became safe havens as I processed all the volatile emotions I constantly experienced. Out there on the field, as part of a team on a mission, I knew exactly what to do and how to do it. The better I got at that, the more relief I felt from the pandemonium throughout the rest of my life. Where my life felt like a sea full of storms, the gym and achievement in sports came to feel like ships that could carry me through it all.

Knowing I had cricket or rugby practice in the afternoon gave me something to look forward to during the day. I saw schoolwork and the social aspects of school as a challenge that I needed to overcome. I did reasonably well in school considering the things that were going on in my home life but the reward for that was always sports at the end of the day. This reward aspect of sport became real for me as, one year, my dad kept me from going on a cricket tour with my team because my school marks were not up to standards. This is something that has stuck with me to this day . . . Ultimately, I made good marks, which contributed to me earning my honors blazer in the eleventh grade. This was given to those who had four colors in four disciplines.

My first three stripes came from becoming an accomplished athlete. During my sophomore year, I made the senior first cricket team, and that same year, I became the only boy in my grade to also make the senior, first rugby team. Then, my junior year, I became the rugby team captain. I also started playing for the junior under nineteen Lions, representing my province of Gauteng (equivalent to playing for your state in the USA) with a partial scholarship that covered my expenses associated with playing the game in college.

I earned my fourth stripe by getting honors for service because I was a prefect—essentially, the head of the senior grade. We were voted in by our fellow students to represent them to the school, and the school picked us to represent the school to our fellow learners. Plus, my classmates voted me deputy head boy, meaning I got to assist as an intermediary between students and school administrators, communicating their needs to each other.

I felt a sense of purpose, stability, and identity through all of this, particularly through the recognition I received from my teammates, classmates, and authority figures. This gave me a heady, powerful feeling sneakily similar to feeling loved. Years would pass before I learned the difference. At the time, however, I felt a deep need for that recognition. I performed well, and in the madness of my life, performing well gave me the consistent praise and respect I craved.

No matter what happened in my personal life, I felt I'd made something of myself in my school, earned a good reputation, and, as a result, found respect and camaraderie with everyone around me. Nothing could take that away from me, no matter what turmoil my family might bring into my life—or so I thought.

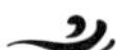

Toward the beginning of matric[4], on the bus ride home from a rugby tournament, my dad phoned me and said, "Listen, you've got to find somewhere else to stay. You can't come home."

I didn't know the details, but from what I pieced together later on, our home and belongings were no longer ours. This was a hugely sad day for me, as I know how hard my dad fought for me and the life we had. For things to get to this point, they must have been bad. I know that must have been an extremely hard phone call for my dad to make.

Apart from the many emotions I felt that evening, I remember just wishing that there was something I could do to help. In many ways, I feel that what came next was that help for him—an ease of the pressure of having me to worry about.

My next phone call went to Jacques's dad, Uncle Kosie. After I explained what was going on, he said, "Ashton, I'm coming to fetch you, and we can talk more when I see you . . . "

4 Senior year in South African high schools.

When we got to their house, we spoke about the situation further. They didn't need much detail or explanation before saying that they would happily have me stay with them.

Where working out and playing sports had been like ships helping me weather the stormy seas of my life, Uncle Kosie and Aunty Josi and their family offered me safe harbor.

You may be thinking . . . What about my mom?

At the time, she had remarried and had another child, my second brother, Trent, whom I love dearly. However, there was a big part of me that didn't feel like her home was mine anymore. At the same time, I was happy for her as she deserved to find happiness and build a family of her own.

Even now, this is difficult for me to write about because I feel there is still a lot of work for me to do to gain clarity around this situation, but the reality was, at that point, it didn't seem financially feasible for her to support me. In addition, there was a big part of me that didn't feel like her home was mine anymore. At the same time, I was happy for her as she deserved to find happiness and build a family of her own. However, I felt very distant to that—an outsider, if you will.

The hardest part came that Christmas. I had been staying with Uncle Kosie and Aunty Josi for most of that year but was visiting my mom for Christmas. At that time, she announced that she was pregnant with my sister, Kendyl, whom I also love and adore to bits.

This was a hard one for me to understand or deal with at the time I felt like a had a lack of financial support from my own mother, yet she was dedicating that support to growing what felt like to me was her "new" family. As much as I want to hold space and show empathy towards my mother for what she was going through, it's also important for me to have self-compassion and understand that my experience was real. It's important that I don't ignore or avoid my experience, including the emotions I felt in that moment. This will be a continuous theme throughout this book. Having gone through the experience of writing this memoir, I find myself experiencing feelings of guilt, questioning myself, and even gaslighting myself in a sense, which has prevented me from being able to process or deal with how certain events in my life have actually affected me. It's an ongoing process, one that I'm still navigating to this day.

Since Uncle Kosie lived in the south of JoBurg and moving in with him would require transferring to the high school in that area, I had to inform various people at my current school. Remember, I was a well liked and influential figure there between my academic and sports-related achievements. So, when I spoke with my principal, she broke down into tears and tried to find a way to keep me there, offering to let me live on campus with one of the teachers. She fought hard to keep me in her house.

I considered it. Once again, I felt pulled in opposing directions. No matter where life took me next, I also seemed required to leave something behind.

The thought of changing schools made me quite emotional. Entering matric, my final year, I'd expected to reap the benefits of my accumulated successes. I'd done so much work and looked forward to representing my school as a leader. I'd accomplished so much there. Switching schools would mean losing much of the camaraderie, respect, and reputation I'd spent four years building. In a way, I felt like I was going from being a hero to being a nobody.

However, being part of a family unit meant more to me than anything else, and I knew that living with Jacques and his parents would give me that. So, I chose to move in with them.

With this came grief. An important part of my life was coming to an end—a part of my life I had truly loved—and I felt that pain in full. In some sense, I had to endure a mourning period during which I grieved the loss of the matric I could have had. At the same time, I also saw benefits to the transition. For all the grief that accompanies change, there exists equal opportunity for joy.

I found it healthy to focus on things outside of my achievements. I'd already demonstrated what I could accomplish, and that's all that really mattered. In addition, this would enable me to finish high school relieved of the responsibility and pressure that came with things like being deputy head boy or captain of the rugby team. Having proven to myself I could earn those things, now I felt I could just finish matric as a normal schoolkid, which may have been the best for me considering what I was going through.

Furthermore, as I began at the new school, I also found joy in the new experience of getting to spend time with some of Jacques's friends, some of whom I'd also known since we were little. Although I missed my old classmates and teammates, new bonds began to form and older bonds deepened, particularly as I began playing rugby at the new school. My reputation on the pitch preceded me a bit, and some of my new teammates knew me from playing against each other over the years. Not only that, but as the new school's administration learned of my situation, they gave me an athletic scholarship. This had the dual benefit of alleviating the financial burden on Uncle Kosie and Aunt Josi while also providing me with a new sense of accomplishment.

Once again, sports supplied me with a figurative ship to weather the turbulence brought on by the new direction life pulled me. I was presented with new challenges, but life was good.

The school year followed in kind. Jacques and I grew closer than ever, sharing a room throughout the year. This gave me a deepened sense of brotherhood with him that I cherished. We even shared a bed, and he's a big guy—taller than six feet. Somehow, we never fought once, not even as our stress reached its max during the intense period of preparing for final exams.

In the end, I had a wonderful year of matric to finish my high school experience. In this, I realized how resilient I was. It became clear to me that no matter how dire a situation seemed at first glance, good things waited for me as long as I looked for them.

Through it all, Uncle Kosie, Aunt Josi, Jacques, and Jacques's two sisters never wavered in providing me that safe harbor. They were my port in the storm. I wanted for nothing with them, from clothes to food to a comfortable bed to love. They treated me as their own, and I truly came to feel like part of their family.

That carried on beyond matric as well, throughout my following three years of varsity. I continued to play rugby and progressed to my highest level yet, playing rugby for money. Unfortunately, this became a different animal. As I struggled with hamstring injuries and a drill sergeant of a coach, I was faced with a decision to push through and see where rugby would take me, or dedicate my focus to building my profession career in the corporate space. Ultimately, I chose the latter.

I continued to work out regularly, and preparing for a life of my own excited me. Not knowing what I really wanted to do, I chose to study for a degree that was broad enough to be applicable across any business: intrapreneurship, a field similar to entrepreneurship but with a focus on using entrepreneurial skills within the context of an established company. As an entrepreneur, I would take on all the risk myself with my own money invested—great risk that can also come with great reward. On the flip side, the concept of intrapreneurship involved essentially operating as an entrepreneur within a business that somebody else had already built or was building. I would find a company to employ me as a creative and would identify new ways to save money, develop products, and perform other tasks of that nature. I would help a company grow and be paid from the profits I helped them gain.

To earn this degree, I studied standard subjects for this field, such as business management, marketing, financial management, human resource management, accounting, economics, and, naturally, entrepreneurship. I still didn't know exactly what I wanted to do, but I knew I wanted to make money and lots of it. This all seemed to point me in that direction.

My second year of varsity, however, life set me on a new and unexpected course. I began working as a bartender, and one evening, my establishment held a ladies' night that featured some male dancers brought in by a company called Pulse International. Around the same time, some friends of mine told me that they knew another way I could make good money on the side—hundreds of rand every night working for just an hour or two—while also having a lot of fun. The work, in short, was to put on a G-string and apron and perform duties such as serving shots to women at bachelorette parties and other events. As it turned out, they were also working for Pulse, the same company that had provided my bar the dancers.

Their exquisite name? The Bare Butt Butlers.

I was intrigued. You got to hang out with people who were partying, show them all a good time, and make some money too? That sounded like the most silly and fantastic job that my twenty-year-old self could have ever imagined.

That's right, ladies and gentlemen—I joined the crew.

# CHAPTER 3

Life as a member of the BBB was more fun than I could have imagined. We attended events of all sizes, donned our G-strings and aprons, and made sure everyone had their drinks and a great time to go with them. After my shift, I often ended up partying with some of them. For a fun-loving twenty-year-old varsity student just looking for all the excitement he could find, I figured I could certainly have a worse job.

At a big health, wellness, and sexuality expo, called SexPo, later that year, the company had me trade in my apron and don faux tuxedo cuffs, half-shirts, and bowties—very Chippendales. I patrolled the event in my alluring attire, handing out drinks and promotional materials for the Pulse Ladies' Lounge after-hours events. During those, a rush of people would fill our lounge, where we would play games and generally give attendees a night to remember.

Pulse also had a production team that put on a big show on a main stage for this event. This show starred professional dancers who performed choreographed routines while disrobing from various costumes such as sailors, firemen, SWAT team members—all sorts of things. These guys were the real hotshots of the show, and hundreds, if not thousands, of people watched them, going wild, having the time of their lives.

In life, one good thing often leads us to a better thing, and this was one such moment. I decided that while I'd been having a grand time with the Bare Butt Butler life, my heart belonged on that stage.

After some discussion with one of the Pulse partners, I scored an invite to their rehearsals, where they gave me a chance to show what I could do. Possessing minimal technical dance skills but limitless energy and enthusiasm, I learned to put on a show. I picked up some of the choreography, found a bit of rhythm, and depended on my body to handle the rest. To my delight, things worked out. Soon, I'd made it onto their team of performers and begun working my way up from smaller bachelorette parties to clubs to even larger shows.

I began to feel like I was living in a bit of a dreamworld. Earning me 500 rand a night, my job consisted of performing a thirty-minute dance routine, then hanging out at the club with everyone I'd just performed for. At this point in the night, we dancers were treated like mini celebrities for a few hours. People gave us drinks, and when we had to pay for our own beverages, we used the money we'd just earned during our performance for these amazing, fun people whom we now got to party with. In my mind, at that time, life could not be better.

All of this brought me full circle, back to SexPo, where I found myself performing on the very stage from the year before. After that performance, while hanging out with one of the Pulse partners, someone invited us to their house to continue partying there, so we exited the venue in search of transportation. Finding a van for hire, we loaded in and took off, striking up a conversation with the driver as we rode. At one point, I asked the driver how he liked this job, just making small talk, and he jokingly acted offended that I thought he was *just* a driver. As it turned out, he owned another entertainment company working the expo. That's how I met Glen, who would become my close friend and one of the most influential people in my life.

In the meantime, however, chaos took hold of my life once again, inexorably pulling me in opposing directions—only this time, unfortunately, this chaos was my own creation.

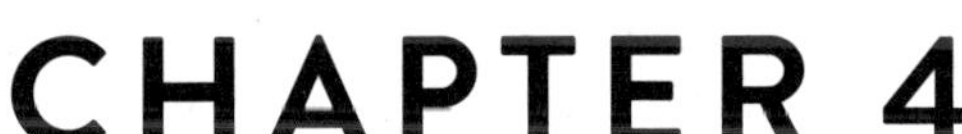

# CHAPTER 4

Leading up to my third year of varsity, I'd been making good marks, so Uncle Kosie and his company offered me a deal. In exchange for sponsoring my final year of varsity, they wanted me to work for them for a few years after I graduated. I accepted the offer, again overwhelmed by gratitude at how Uncle Kosie continued to serve as this safe harbor in my life. Not only had he continued to provide me with food and shelter beyond high school, but now he had helped to secure me a career steppingstone.

In all my experience, I've found that security and safety come not from the place we live or even the circumstances of our lives but more so from the people we live with. Of course, the most important person we live with our entire lives is ourselves, and it would take me quite some time to find security and safety within myself.

Upon graduation, I began working at Uncle Kosie's company as a junior verification analyst, a role in which I assisted in auditing our clients' business practices in accordance with South African Black Economic Empowerment policies. At the same time, I continued to make money dancing on the side.

This combination worked well for me. With Uncle Kosie's company, I began building the corporate career I'd been told I needed to make my way in the world, even if the work felt somewhat boring for me. A standard nine-to-five job, it required me to gather and review paperwork all day, examine whether businesses were in compliance with regulations, and communicate my findings to my bosses and our clients. Useful and valuable work, of course—just a bit more tedious than what came naturally to me. I craved stimulation, and my dancing with Pulse provided that. I could still have fun, experience new things, and party, all while generating a decent supplemental income.

Soon enough, however, that became an issue with my new bosses. They expressed concern that I might end up dancing for someone their clients knew on a weekend and then find myself in meetings with said clients the next week. For obvious reasons, that would be a bit uncomfortable, if not outright unprofessional. Ultimately, my bosses told me to make a decision: either truly start my career and focus on my job with their company per our agreement or break our agreement and continue to be a dancer. I could not do both.

Again, I felt pulled between two forces. However, recognizing this as a moment when I must choose to be responsible and mature, I told them that I understood their position, and I stopped dancing and focused on giving my new job my full attention.

From that point forward, I entrenched myself in that work. Without dancing to offer extra income, I focused on making as much money as I could as quickly as I could. I'd wake up at 6 a.m., work out, eat breakfast, put on my dress shirt, and be in the office by eight every morning. My world became one of spreadsheets and paperwork and reports.

Before long, I earned a promotion from junior verification analyst to senior verification analyst, at which point my job offered some exciting potential. The harder I worked and the more I trained other junior verification analysts, the more money I could make. The company presented a clear structure of how I could maximize my earnings by finding more clients to bring into the business and by training other auditors to report to me.

As this unfolded, my friend Dave and I decided to buy a house together. We'd known each other since we were kids, having met through Jacques, and he'd always been around Jacques's family, too, while we were growing up. After living together in a university hostel and then graduating around the same time, we decided that becoming roommates and co-owners on a house would work out to be an ideal situation.

After a bit of searching, we made our purchase: a brick townhome with three bedrooms and two bathrooms, two floors, and even an outdoor deck that included a braai area and a jacuzzi. I threw a mattress down on my bedroom floor, and we furnished the community areas with the absolute bare minimum. I provided an old refrigerator and cabinet that doubled as a TV stand, while Dave got his hands on an old, beaten-up couch with deep red leather, odd wood legs, and other trappings.

We loved that place. A milestone for me, that house represented the manifestation of my independence and self-reliance and gave me such gratitude and joy every time I returned home. I felt I had attained a new level of success in life.

Of course, each new level we reach in life shifts the spotlight to the next level we need to reach. So, throwing myself into my work, as well as buying that house with Dave, only revealed new ways in which I needed to grow. I was proud of my accomplishments, but I wasn't satisfied. I wanted to maintain that forward (and upward) momentum.

Growing up in a family that constantly struggled financially—and especially seeing my father lose everything, including our home, due to money issues—had left me with a deep desire to generate my own income. Now I was, and the more money I made, the more I wanted to make. Over time, I built a solid team that worked with me, earning commissions that also earned me extra income. Following the company's structure, my hard work began to pay off very well for me as well as those working under me. My salary and commissions added up to as much as 30,000 to 40,000 rand some months, which felt like a remarkable amount of money to me at that young age.

Things were going so well, in fact, that I started to feel sort of nervous. I'm not sure how much sense this makes, but I began to feel afraid of my success—uncomfortable perhaps. With wonderful friends, ongoing love and support from Uncle Kosie and Auntie Josi, close bonds with Jacques and his sisters, and my excellent income to boot, everything in my life pointed in the right direction. Things were going so well that I almost expected something bad to happen soon—and then, I ended up being the reason something bad *did* happen.

Around this time, I became impatient in my pursuit of making more money, and in my impatience, I made some bad decisions. Due to the sensitivity of the situation, I'm going to spare the details. The short and simple version of the story is that I made unethical business deals for myself that negatively impacted my relationship with Jacques, Uncle Kosie, and the entire family.

One day, Jacques appeared in my office and told me that they knew everything. Instantly, my body went cold, and my brain collapsed into anxiety-riddled paralysis.

You know the way it feels to be in a dark room and then the lights suddenly come on? That pain and disorientation? That's how this felt. The lights had been off because I didn't want to see the mess I was making. Then, the switch was thrown, and I had no choice but to look.

My best friend and his family had taken care of me for five years prior to this, starting when I had nowhere else to go. They'd gone on to offer me this position in their company to help advance my career. And after all that, I went behind their backs, took advantage of their kindness, and did irreparable harm to their hearts and our relationship.

The conversations to follow with Uncle Kosie, Aunty Josi, and Jacques' sisters were probably the most uncomfortable conversations I have ever had. I felt small, broken, and unworthy of the family I always wanted.

To this day, this situation—the shame and the guilt—haunts me. I continue to think about and try to figure out what it was that allowed me to go through with something that would cause so much destruction to everything that I valued so much. There was something in me that deliberately avoided and ignored every bit of character, sincerity, discipline, and honor I possessed. Some part of me that I struggle to own.

Depression set in, and I felt very lost and alone. Many times in my life, when faced with adversity, I could easily just get on with it and do what I needed to do, but this time, it was different. I struggled to find direction or purpose. The flame of burning desire that had always burnt so strong in me was just about dead—smothered in shame.

Things changed at work too, as I really started questioning what I wanted to do with my life. It had been really convenient for me to walk straight into a job from college. I'd been able to buy my own house, and it had allowed me the financial independence I so badly wanted. In most ways, I was an independent young adult, but I was beginning to see that I just was not cut out for the corporate world.

Meanwhile, the company underwent some unrelated changes. One day, our bosses called us down to the boardroom where they told us that our compensation structure was changing. Going forward, we would no longer earn commissions off people we brought into the business, nor would we be given a share of the profits generated by employees whom we trained and managed.

At around twenty-five years old at this point, I'd spent two or three years developing a good reputation among clients as well as building a team of verification analysts working underneath me. I had worked hard in myriad legitimate ways to capitalize on the company's established commission and benefits structure. Now, with these changes, they eradicated all I stood to gain from what I had built there.

Surrounded by papers and files, I constantly found myself day-dreaming about what my dancing friends might be doing. Since I stayed in touch with some of them and saw them once in a while, I knew about gigs they were working and the awesome places they were traveling to. Hearing about big events where they performed brought back a lot of good memories and made me crave that sense of excitement and adventure again.

Meanwhile, there I sat in my office, wearing my professional shirt and tie, which were quite different from those I'd worn while dancing, and just lacking the incentive to work hard that had once so motivated me. All I had to do was tediously check other companies' calculations, examine the evidence they'd provided to support their calculations, and file reports about how said evidence did or did not, in fact, support said calculations. I did this day after day after day.

I felt a sense of decay inside me, like how you see leaves and branches withering on plants beginning to rot. But I chose to see this perceived negative situation as a change of seasons. These leaves needed to fall off and decay into the earth, only to create nutrients so that during the next season, new colorful and lively leaves could grow again.

Clearly, I was made for other work. Having tasted another lifestyle, one of making a living through performing and working a schedule that offered new challenges and experiences every day, I became increasingly disenchanted with my current role. Even though I knew that I would never make a career as a professional dancer, I was convinced that by changing my environment, I would be exposed to opportunities along the way. Who knows what could happen?

Feeling drawn back toward that world, I began to spend more time with Glen and others I'd previously met through dancing. In so doing, I began to party with them again, and that ultimately led to a life-changing epiphany.

# CHAPTER 5

One Thursday night, Glen and I went to one of our regular spots, a bar in a big casino and hotel complex, and we ended up staying out until three in the morning. A few hours later, we made our way into work, hungover, possibly still intoxicated, and wearing the same clothes as the day before. We'd had such a great night that we decided to do it again the next week. And then, we did it again the week after that. More friends joined us each time, and we ended up christening this new tradition as The Thursday Club.

In time, The Thursday Club evolved to the point where, immediately after work on Friday, I met back up with Glen and some mates to continue partying at different bars and clubs. Then, on Saturday mornings, despite the inevitable hangovers, we powered through, finding more ways to party the day away. All of this progressed until the partying would carry on through Sunday as well, the weekends becoming one big cycle of bars and casinos and dance clubs and house parties.

Some weekends, we'd go to a music festival. Other weekends, we'd spontaneously pile into a couple of cars and drive three hours to Sun City, a massive world-renowned resort that's part wave park, part casino and golf course, where we'd live it up for two or three days straight.

As the partying consumed more and more of my time, I began some workweeks by walking into the office on Monday morning still a bit drunk from the night before.

With all this going on, I felt caught between these two worlds. In one, I had a solid, respectable corporate job that didn't bring me any joy anymore. In the other, I had the entertainment and partying I loved but also felt that chipping away at my productivity in my job. Yet again, I found myself being pulled in separate directions, needing to let go of one in order to make the most of the other.

I realized that, despite everything happening at the company—the mistakes I'd made, the changing structure affecting my income—my core issue was that I couldn't see how, if I remained there, I could continue to grow. The more time went on, the more I wanted to leave that job.

For a while, I battled with guilt over this. For many years, Uncle Kosie had been loving and loyal toward me without fail, and I felt tremendous gratitude for all that he had done for me. In some sense, I felt I owed him and his company my loyalty in return. On the other hand, I didn't want to be loyal to them to the detriment of my career, and I felt that I needed to do what was best for myself too.

One day, I phoned Glen and asked him if I could work for him at his company, which I'll call Fresh Productions. He and his partner worked out a deal for me to be hired on as a production assistant.

As that fell into place, I decided to resign from the auditing job at Uncle Kosie's company. Entering into that conversation, I felt anxious and sad, but in his typical fashion, Uncle Kosie responded with nothing but grace and kindness. He said that he understood and that he wanted to support me however he could, even if that meant I needed to try something else for my career. No matter what, he told me, he would always be there for me.

In short, Fresh was an "entertainment solutions" company that provided entertainment for various events. For example, we would do the year-end corporate party for Cell C[5], supplying them with a dozen dancers in outfits with props on a stage. We always put on a proper production to the delight of our clients and audience. Glen would handle the production side of things, his partner was the creative director and choreographer, and I served as the utility guy, doing anything that they needed me to do. Sometimes, I even danced again.

Still in my mid-twenties, I didn't really know where my life was going at this point, but I knew that I needed this lifestyle—for the time being, at least. The thrill the work gave me felt like breathing fresh air for the first time in a long time. Some days, I'd wake up at 9 or 10 a.m., start working around noon or 1 p.m., then work until 2 or 3 a.m. The ever-changing schedule suited me much more than my standard nine-to-five schedule had. Waking up at 6 a.m., hitting the gym, going to work, coming home, eating, going to bed, rinsing, repeating, day after day—that had bored me nearly to tears. Now, I had an admittedly chaotic schedule that kept me on my toes—invigorated and engaged.

Working with Fresh every day gave me the stimulation I'd craved. The people in the event and entertainment industry felt like my kind of people, cut from a different cloth with a vibrant energy about them. This job was never dull. Although I knew I wouldn't be here forever and viewed the experience as transitional instead of career building, I focused on simply enjoying the ride.

I began dancing a bit more for Fresh again whenever I could, sometimes getting paid as much for two stage shows as I was paid for all the other work I was doing. As I continued seeking growth and expansion, I began doing some sales for Fresh too. Eventually, I also helped them run their new promotional division alongside my girlfriend at the time, Nikita, a dancer and wardrobe manager for the company.

---

5 One of South Africa's larger cell phone networks, similar to AT&T in the States.

We traveled around South Africa to cities like Durban and Cape Town, where I did mainstage shows as well as promotional work at bars and casinos. Often, I dressed up to provide extra entertainment at events, sometimes performing as a Chippendales dancer, other times donning elaborate costumes. At a Valentine's Day event, I appeared as a giant heart. For an Easter event, I became a giant bunny, climbing onto some stilts and dancing like that all over the place. Nikita even helped me create some original costumes, such as a twelve-foot hexabot light outfit that went nearly a story and a half high.

My job became about just making people happy. Sometimes in life, we have those seasons that require us to simply have fun doing what we're doing, both for healing and for escape. That's what this job gave me.

# CHAPTER 6

While training at a CrossFit gym, I became friends with a man I'll call Rory. At some point, Rory asked if I'd like to come work for him. He ran a company that we can refer to as Bounce. Similar to Fresh, Bounce intrigued me because of its larger, more corporate structure, meaning there was more opportunity for growth in my career.

The timing proved serendipitous too. Without going into detail, Fresh had begun experiencing some various instabilities that had become increasingly frustrating. I didn't want to go back to a job as a corporate paper-pusher, but I also hoped to find a role with a bit more security than Fresh could provide. As I spoke with Rory, I realized Bounce offered exactly that.

So, after thanking Glen for everything, I made the move to Bounce. Sometimes, I realized, growth means leaving something behind.

As with all things in my life, I dove into my work at Bounce headfirst. A brand activation and outdoor media advertising agency, Bounce needed me to serve as a client service and sales manager. I came up with marketing strategies for brands, which required duties such as interactive marketing, in-store promotions, road shows, and anything else engaging the end consumers face to face. This was called below-the-line advertising, which we combined with above-the-line advertising in print, television, radio, and billboards. We operated in territories all across the African continent.

For instance, a food corporation client would invent new flavors for their products and task us with developing creative ways to introduce those new flavors into markets. We often focused our efforts on township-like areas known as "the kasi." Instead of just going into malls and putting up signs and handing out samples, we became part of the kasi's culture.

Rory and the Bounce business partners took me under their wing, even including me in meetings. This enabled me to start coming into my own as I cultivated a better understanding of the business and discovered how to become more confident and comfortable as I worked with clients.

There was a lot to learn. As client service and sales manager, I developed concepts, presented those concepts to clients in hopes of convincing them to approve more budget for us, and then executed the concepts that they approved.

The work kept me driven and focused. With a small salary complemented by heavy commission-based incentives, I could once again earn more for working harder and smarter. House accounts provided nice, small commissions, and if I persuaded them to spend more budget with us, I earned commissions from that too.

For example, the food company had a sizable marketing budget that they spent on us as well as two or three additional marketing companies. However, we could pitch them concepts that could net us more of their budget. Put a different way, we could fight for bigger slices of the pie. Should my pitch be one that did just that, then I'd be rewarded in kind.

Bounce also offered substantial increases in compensation to motivate me to go out hunting for bigger clients that could translate into greater sales. In other words, the more I grew in this position, the more money I could make. This sort of structure suited my personality well, and I began to find real success, landing big accounts from new clients and convincing them to spend big budgets with Bounce.

For the first time in my life, I started earning truly substantial money. Some months, I made nearly 100,000 rand. For a point of reference, the bond on my house with David might have been around 9,000 rand, and my car payment might have been around 5,000 rand. Making 100,000 rand per month put me in fantastic financial shape. To reward myself, I bought a motocross bike, sold my little Volkswagen car, and purchased a BMW.

I also partied like money was no object. In fact, around this time, I began going a bit wild. I'd also become friends with some of Rory's business partners, riding bikes with one on one day, partying with another the next day, then all coming together to party on yet another day.

Somewhere over the course of this phase of my life, I earned myself the delightful nickname of "Smashton," or "Smash" for short. A term of endearment bestowed upon me by my partying brethren and sistren, Smashton became like my fun-loving alter-ego, a person I became once I reached a certain level of intoxication. In many ways, he was my favorite version of myself, the life of every party and wholly confident in his own skin.

Despite the fact that I'd been an adult dancer and, before that, an athlete and prominent member of my school's student body, I was actually a rather shy person by nature. Simply standing around in a bar, engaging in small talk or making friends, didn't come as naturally to me as you might assume—at least, until I got a few drinks in me. Then, Smashton emerged, and suddenly, nobody was a stranger. Everybody was a potential lifelong best mate. I felt self-assured and gave no shits what anybody else thought. I danced, I sang, and I loved everything and everyone around me in full and without condition.

In many ways, I wished I could be more like Smashton when I was sober because sober Ashton was reserved and anxious in ways that might have surprised people who knew me well. One of my goals was to find a way to feel more like Smashton when I was not under the influence of alcohol.

In the meantime, Smashton was living life to the fullest. When partying until four or five in the morning, my only limit seemed to be the sunrise. Once I saw the horizon start to turn from black to that hazy yellow and orange, and I heard the birds start to sing, I suddenly felt an overpowering, occasionally disgusted, urge to dive onto the nearest bed or couch. Something about knowing I'd spent my entire night partying until the sun came up made me feel a bit sick of myself.

Nevertheless, we'd wake up the next day and start it up all over again. We all had a classic young man's work hard, play hard approach to life, and sometimes, we played harder than we worked. Then, we'd go work hard again to balance the scales.

All of that happened with just one of my groups of friends. I had another group of friends who also loved to party, and I usually met up with them after living it up with my work friends half the weekend. Again, Friday night rolled into Saturday afternoon rolled into Sunday night, and some weekends, the party didn't stop until Monday morning. I'd go into work on Monday, endure until I could properly function, and then work hard to balance it all out.

After all, I've always embraced a good challenge. In this case, I created the challenge for myself every week. As someone who thrives on being constantly on the move, I juggled everything well—for a while. However, in time, it began catching up with me.

The primary issue, I discovered, was the inconsistent nature of the pay. I might make a significant amount a few months out of the year, but other months, my income might be much lower. In addition, living this rockstar sort of lifestyle, I started to feel like a wreck. Many workweeks started with hangovers. Yet every Thursday and Friday, I felt the irresistible pull to party again, constantly in search of the next thrill—the next party, the next girl, the next high.

With all that I was doing, I spent all my money. Having never learned to adhere to a personal budget, build savings, or anything of that nature, I burned through all my funds almost as soon as they came in. Perhaps it was reckless and irresponsible, but I was living in the moment and just having fun, consumed by a need for constant stimulation.

To my surprise, after some time, this routine started to feel old. I began to grow tired of the partying and the drinking. I felt caught in a loop of searching for stimulation. This undermined my sense of control.

Even partying becomes boring when that's all you do to fill your life.

Plus, on occasion, a night of drinking and partying could take an unfortunate turn, resulting in a blowout of some sort. Smashton was all fun and games and love until, one or two nights a year, he wasn't. Something would happen, I would become emotional and angry, and that would lead to some sort of commotion or even a full-blown fight. After drinking to a certain point, somebody might make a comment or take an action that would set something off in me that I didn't understand but that I felt with overwhelming force, as though something had been boiling inside of me without me even realizing it. Then, I would explode.

For example, one night, I returned home from partying and smelled marijuana in the house. As it turned out, Dave had been smoking weed inside, which I'd been strongly against. I never liked weed, and I *really* didn't like the smell of it, so I'd tried to establish a rule that we wouldn't smoke weed in the house.

Dave and I had butted heads over this a couple of times before, and for whatever reason, on this night, I just ran out of patience. Since he had been partying, too, and we were both drunk, we quickly found ourselves in an intense confrontation. He thought I was overreacting, and I thought he was being inconsiderate. There's no other way to say this: I lost my shit. We ended up in a nearly full-scale physical altercation, and things escalated to the point that I put my elbow through his bedroom door.

Although that was one of our more volatile exchanges, such aggressive confrontations happened on occasion, and a couple of times a year, I would have a blowout like that either at home or out at a club somewhere. Usually, these instances coincided with times when I was experiencing a lot of other stress elsewhere in my life. I'd go out drinking and partying to escape it and find myself triggered by someone over the course of the night. Emotionally immature, I would feel tension and frustration build up to a boiling point until I struck a wall or a door or something to release that pent-up emotion. When the physical blow made me feel pain in my body, that had a way of snapping me out of the tension that had built up. But by then, the momentary damage was done.

Dave handled the situation at our house with grace, though, always the more level-headed one between the two of us and never one to take things personally or stand in judgment of someone's worse moments. He knew me well enough to know I never meant him any harm, and he accepted my apology the next day. Soon enough, we were laughing about the whole situation, and I replaced the door as soon as I could.

I knew that sort of behavior was not okay, but Dave never judged me for it or made me feel like there was something inherently wrong with me. He supported me through what I was going through, and his understanding and kindness during my worse moments enabled me to grow into a more emotionally intelligent person. He loved and accepted Ashton and Smashton, and that helped me begin to do the same.

Even still, I started to feel lost as my life spiraled into what felt like a series of weeks full of chaos. I wanted to find a way to better understand both Ashton and Smashton and figure out how to merge the two. That way, I could be carefree and secure without relying so much on alcohol, and I wouldn't be at risk of losing my shit in full Smashton mode. With no true path to follow in my pursuit of this idealized version of myself, however, I needed a clearer sense of direction, so I went searching for it.

Having remained friends with Glen, we spoke often, and he always had a way of remaining practical about any situation. He maintained an uncanny ability to view circumstances from multiple perspectives in a way I aspired to emulate. During our conversations, Glen would often say profound things that resonated with me in meaningful and significant fashion.

For example, one day, while talking with him on the phone about how disorganized and confusing my life often felt, he told me, "Your outside world is a reflection of your inside world." I was instantly struck by the power and truth of this statement.

Wanting to learn more from Glen, I asked him for some resources that had taught him his most valuable lessons. In response, Glen gave me some DVDs of human behavioral specialist Dr. John DeMartini, which included one talk titled "Balancing Emotions." In this talk, Dr. DeMartini described ways to understand our emotions, values, behaviors, and painful memories and how to navigate our traumatic experiences in order to stop them from ruling our lives.

To recap his entire presentation would require several dozen pages of this book, but perhaps the most simple and impactful way for me to distill what I learned from it is this: You attract what you feel. If you feel worried and fearful, you attract opportunities to fulfill your worries and fears. If you feel chaotic, you attract a life that brings you more chaos. And if you are confident and calm and at peace, regardless of the circumstances you face in your life, you attract opportunities to create more good things that further enhance your confidence and peace.

One of the most memorable lessons from that talk was on what Dr. DeMartini called "the implicate order of the universe." After describing the makeup of the universe down to the molecular structure of an atom, he made the point that in every aspect of life, there will always exist a positive and a negative. From our relationships to our careers to anything else we might do with our lives, we will always experience a negative to balance out a positive and vice versa. Where good happens, bad will follow, and where bad happens, good will follow—so don't get too high on the good, and don't be too disappointed by the bad. "Just expect it," Dr. DeMartini said. "That's just the implicate order of the universe."

Sometimes, the positive or negative of a situation depends on the way you experience it, which has to do with other factors DeMartini discussed. For example, he taught me that people will always act according to their values, meaning there is power in understanding that other people will always have a different perspective than you. Relative to that, he also discussed the emotional charges we attach to circumstances, which again relates to our perception of them and can determine how positive or negative the situation actually is for us. Part of dealing with our emotions and our traumas, I learned, is finding the roots of the emotional charge we associate with them.

I had no idea just how relevant all of this would become over the next few years of my life, but even in the beginning, this talk deeply resonated with me. I must have listened to it twenty times. My mind felt opened by this revelation, providing a new foundation for me in my growing hunger to learn and evolve.

Next, I attended a course workshop called TAG, which stands for "Think Act Grow." Based on the speaker's personal experiences combined with teachings from Napoleon Hill's book *Think and Grow Rich,* this course helped me become more honest with myself. I realized that I'd been making excuses for why I couldn't do certain things in my life. See, the course explored the ways that we want to blame our circumstances on matters that are supposedly out of our control—and the ways that we can take extreme accountability and responsibility for our lives. Nobody else will make the things I want happen for me. I have to make them happen myself.

To show me how, the course took me deeper into the power of the subconscious mind, introducing me to concepts that I'd never heard of before. It guided me to think of the mind like a Ferrari—an amazing vehicle but one you must still properly learn how to operate. Ferraris are exquisitely designed masterpieces of aerodynamics and performance with massive engines. But drive one without understanding it, and you can easily crash.

Between Dr. DeMartini's talks and this TAG course, I was discovering just how much control I really had over myself. With a dawning sense of enlightenment and empowerment, I began to realize I simply needed to learn how to better manage my mind to prevent myself from crashing.

The key to all of this was a concept called radical accountability: being completely honest about the role I played in everything that happened to me. Nobody was going to show up and lay out the way for me to live a personally fulfilling life. I was the only one who could do that. So, I also came to think of radical accountability as *extreme responsibility.*

Of course, we can't control harmful choices others make or unfortunate circumstances that might affect us. Radical accountability isn't about magical thinking. It's not pretending that bad things don't feel bad to experience or that they don't potentially have devastating consequences. Rather, radical accountability means also accepting that we do have control over the mindset with which we meet such challenges and the actions we choose to take after they arise.

For instance, I had to take the time to process my emotions rather than simply reacting to them. When I felt bored, instead of going out partying, I considered that I should take time to understand where that feeling of boredom came from. What parts of my life were lacking, leaving me feeling dissatisfied?

To this end, the TAG course also taught me some basic meditation techniques that helped me work on better understanding my mind and the sources of my emotions. Ultimately, the primary way to bolster my ability to make strong and healthy decisions moving forward was to build up my subconscious mind and train it to work in ways that helped me pursue what I truly wanted in life.

Working hand in hand with radical accountability was another concept TAG taught me: auto-suggestion. Basically, your brain operates similar to a computer, processing information and filing away patterns based on everything fed into it through your senses. This ultimately produces your mind, the connection that exists between your brain and your body. Since your subconscious mind operates as the creative force in your body and your life, what you're putting into your conscious mind will be processed by your subconscious. The thoughts and emotions that you allow yourself to dwell on will become more engrained in your subconscious, which will then become trained to seek out experiences that further reflect what you've been dwelling on. Auto-suggestion means consciously feeding healthy and productive thoughts into your brain to then produce a healthier and more helpful mind. (See how that also connects to what I learned from Dr. DeMartini?)

To assist with this, the course taught us two creeds to memorize verbatim. The first was a modified version of a letter about being a man that Rudyard Kipling once wrote to his son. The second was called the Creed of Attainment. I've included them on the following pages for your convenience in reading and revisiting later.

## KIPLING LETTER ON BEING A MAN

If I can keep my head when all around me
Are losing theirs and blaming it on me,
If I can trust myself when all men doubt me,
But make allowance for their doubting too;
If I can wait and not be tired by waiting,
Or being lied about, don't deal in lies,
Or being hated, don't give way to hating,
And yet don't look too good, nor talk too wise
If I can dream—and not make dreams your master;
If I can think—and not make thoughts my aim;
If I can meet with Triumph and Disaster
And treat those two impostors just the same;
If I can bear to hear the truth I've spoken
Twisted by knaves to make a trap for fools,
Or watch the things I gave my life to, broken,
And stoop and build 'em up with worn-out tools
If I can make one heap of all my winnings
And risk it on one turn of pitch-and-toss,
And lose, and start again at your beginnings
And never breathe a word about my loss;
If I can force my heart and nerve and sinew
To serve my turn long after they are gone,
And so hold on when there is nothing in me
Except the will which says to them: 'Hold on!'
If I can talk with crowds and keep my virtue,
Or walk with Kings — nor lose the common touch,
If neither foes nor loving friends can hurt me,
If all men count with me, but none too much;
If I can fill the unforgiving minute
With sixty seconds' worth of distance run,
Mine is the Earth and everything that's in it,
And—which is more—I'll be a man.

## THE CREED OF ATTAINMENT

I must awake to my true self only by knowing myself when I know all men.

I must take control of my attitude by mastering my thoughts, and I hear and promise to do so.

My right request will attract the right response.

Therefore, I will direct my thoughts for ten minutes daily on picturing the perfect end result of my desires.

Knowing that I will give that my all will give me the courage to live my step-by-step plan with persistence.

My mind can only hold one thought at a time.

Therefore, through the principle of auto suggestion, I'll concentrate my thoughts for 30 minutes daily on directing my energy towards self-understanding.

I realize that to live with truth is to live without fear.

Therefore, I will eliminate all negative thoughts and actions and concentrate on owning myself and living my own life.

I will learn how to be my own best friend, accepting full responsibility for myself and my actions.

I will attract others to me by developing a love for myself and for all humanity, because I know that I cannot expect others to love or respect me if I do not love and respect myself.

I will take part in no transaction unless built in truth, because truth is eternal, pure, and the only power.

Truth will set me free.

Understand that I will receive from life in direct proportion to that which I give to it.

And I promise to give my best.

I'll sign my name to this creed, commit it to memory, and repeat it aloud twice daily, knowing in full faith that it will affect my thoughts, words, and deeds, and that I will become a modest, self-reliant, and successful person.

Having taken the concepts I learned from Dr. DeMartini and the TAG workshop to heart, I began to notice an immediate change in myself.

One of the first nights I went out after the workshop, I attended a concert with some of my friends. When we began partying like usual, I felt like I didn't really belong anymore. All of the partying I'd been doing had been like trying to scratch an itch I just couldn't reach. Now, that version of myself felt obsolete. It was somebody else I no longer was.

I felt as though this workshop pointed me toward the next level of my life and gave me the tools I needed to reach it. By learning more about the mind and, ultimately, myself, I realized how unhappy I had been for a long time and was finally able to recognize that I'd been constantly chasing stimulation as a distraction from that unhappiness.

Around this time, I read Tim Ferriss's *The 4-Hour Work Week*, a book about how to quit your day job and build a career that supports a life you want to live. The concept I took from that book was that most people postpone actually living until they retire, spending 90 percent of their lives working to enjoy just the 10 percent that's left—and that it was possible to flip that on its head. Ferriss laid out the actionable steps he had taken to do that for himself, and his story gave me more confidence and motivation to stop looking at my nine-to-five job as the security in my life.

That, combined with everything else I was learning, helped me change the way I viewed myself and the potential my life held. I just didn't know how to get there. Sitting in my office, I'd begun to find myself spiraling into boredom again. I'd catch myself wondering what else the future held for me and what else I needed to thrive. I felt pulled to travel and see more of the world, party less, learn more, and spend more time in nature and beautiful places. As I became more honest with myself, I realized that I needed more out of life than what I currently had.

However, although *The 4-Hour Work Week* compelled me to strike off on my own, and the lessons from Dr. DeMartini and TAG taught me to believe in myself and use the power of my subconscious to trust in my ability to create a life I wanted for myself, I still felt a need to remain in my job. Bounce had given me an opportunity that meant a great deal to me, and working for them had helped me through a challenging time in my life, so I felt guilty for wanting more than what they had to offer.

Maybe, I thought, I could find what I wanted while remaining at the company. With that in mind, I spoke with Rory and the partners at Bounce about starting an office in Cape Town. That was far enough away to feel fresh and new for me. Plus, it was a very different type of city. Johannesburg is essentially a metropolis, while Cape Town is quite scenic and beautiful with mountains and the beach. The only problem was a lack of opportunity to make real money—and Bounce had no interest in opening an office there.

One day, I found myself standing at the urinal in the restroom at the office, staring out a window in the wall that overlooked a gas station across the street, watching people come and go, feeling an overwhelming need to leave. I couldn't escape the sense that I was like a prisoner in the life I'd made for myself. And a thought entered my mind: *Maybe I should just resign.*

That was a wild concept. How could I do that? I had no other job lined up and no clear idea of where I would go if I *did* resign. Even still, I felt so frustrated, desperately wanting to leave Johannesburg but having no opportunities within Bounce to go anywhere else.

When I was speaking with Glen about this on the phone later, he told me that I was trying to get the best of both worlds. "If you're going to live your life with one foot in two boats," he said, "you'll spend your life never really going in any direction."

In one boat, I had the security and predictability of this job at Bounce and this life in Johannesburg. I might have been frustrated, but I knew what to expect. In the other boat, I didn't know what sort of job I'd have or where I'd go, but I'd be free to pursue a life that felt better and freer than the job at Bounce and my life in Johannesburg could offer me.

"You need to put two feet in one boat," Glen reflected firmly.

As I weighed my options, I considered searching for other jobs while I continued working for Bounce. The notion of just resigning without any sort of backup plan felt daunting to say the least. I had no spouse to support me, and I knew my savings wouldn't last forever. Yet, at the same time, the lessons I'd learned lately filled me with new confidence. By believing in myself to find a way forward, I had faith that things would work out one way or another and that where I might need help, I would find it. As a result, my focus shifted away from a fear of what might go wrong and toward letting go of all the things in life that were not serving me. In making this mental shift, I chose to pursue only that which would contribute to me becoming a better, healthier person.

With that in mind, the boat in which I needed to plant both of my feet became clear: I needed to leave Johannesburg and find a new life somewhere else. In arriving at that conclusion, I calmly and fearlessly noted everything else that would entail. Then, determined to put all my energy into making this next move for my life, I went to Rory, thanked him for the opportunity Bounce had provided me, and told him that I needed to resign.

This decision made no logical sense, of course. At twenty-seven years old, I was leaving my position with no other job lined up and with no clear sense of where I was going to find a new job. My only plan, if you could even call it that, was to sell all my belongings in order to start a new life somewhere else. I had no idea where that new life was going to take me or how I would support myself. All I knew for certain was that I could not stay where I was, and in the wake of all I'd just learned from Dr. DeMartini, the TAG workshop, and more, I could not afford to live in fear. These people were telling me that I had more control over my life than I believed, and I wanted to find out just how true that was.

I believed that something *more*—something that I could pour my heart and soul into—waited for me *out there* in the world. I could feel it, and I believed in myself to find it. To do that, however, I just knew that I had to let go of what I was holding onto first.

I'd finally put both of my feet into one boat.

# CHAPTER 7

After resigning, I spent my mornings at a nearby café, enjoying breakfast and coffee while updating my CV. At the same time, I researched companies and agencies that could offer me a job wherever I might go next. Dubai quickly became my primary focus. I'd heard a lot about how cool of a place it was, and I could go there as an ex-pat and find a job that would pay me in American dollars. So, I applied to fifty or sixty companies and even included a PowerPoint presentation with my CV in an effort to stand out.

As I waited to hear back, I settled into my newfound confidence and further embraced the concept of letting go of things that didn't serve my new mission to become a better, healthier person. As the days and then weeks passed by without any meaningful responses to my job applications, I remained calm and free of anxiety. Despite my unemployment, dwindling savings account, and completely uncertain future, I felt peace. I knew I was making decisions that felt good and true to what I most needed.

To that end, instead of spending my nights on partying and my days on recovering from hangovers, I reduced my drinking, ate and slept well, and devoted my mornings to my job search while patronizing the café. Most afternoons, I began driving some ten minutes outside of the city to visit the Walter Sisulu National Botanical Garden. Located on nature reserves full of hundreds of species of plants, the gardens are part of the Cradle of Humankind, where the first humans were said to have lived. Hiking trails immersed me in lush surroundings, giving me an ideal place to escape the clutter and noise of the city.

One of my favorite locations in the gardens contained a beautiful waterfall where I'd sit in my small, foldable camping chair; remove my socks and shoes; and sink my feet into the verdant grass and cool earth. For hours, I would sit and read and write. Using the new surroundings to inspire new ways of thought, I'd draw on the lessons from Dr. DeMartini and the TAG course to better understand the ways my subconscious mind had impacted me thus far. Along with that, I endeavored to further give my subconscious mind positive and healthy material to use. To this end, I journaled deeply about past experiences, seeking to peel away layers from my upbringing and social conditioning—and separate who I thought I was supposed to be from who I believed I really was.

As much as I wanted to experience profound epiphanies right away in those early days, most of what I journaled was essentially acknowledging that my childhood and subsequent conditioning by society had likely affected me in significant ways—but I was unable to see specifically *how* just yet. That wouldn't come until later. Even still, simply acknowledging those things on paper gave me a sense of tranquility about them and set me on a path to exploring them—a path that would yield shocking and transformative results years later.

In the meantime, I also sought to continue filling my subconscious mind with useful material and discovered a gold mine in Deepak Chopra's audiobook for *The Seven Spiritual Laws of Success.* I was struck by the way he explained how most people live with two masks: our social mask that shows who we want people to think we are and our true mask, which shows who we *really* are. I found it so strange to think about how there can be such huge differences between those two masks and how we, as human beings, can get stuck in trying to present a certain version of ourselves that we think others will love and accept. Meanwhile, we neglect putting time and energy into building up who we truly are.

The most impactful part of the book came in the sixth chapter where he describes The Law of Detachment: "Allow yourself and others the freedom to be who they are. Do not force solutions—allow them to spontaneously emerge. Uncertainty is essential and your path to freedom." Basically, you don't give up your intention or your desire, but you detach from any specific, expected result. Chopra goes on to say this: "The need for security is based on not knowing the true self. Those who seek security chase it for a lifetime without ever finding it."

I felt as though the universe were pushing me into learning exactly how to become comfortable without security. Chopra's words seemed powerful and relevant in light of what happened next: Despite all the CVs and job applications that I'd sent out, I heard almost nothing in return.

As I continued reading Chopra's book, journaling, and meditating, a phrase began to take shape in my mind: *Find security in the unknown.* I wrote it down, and it played on repeat in my head, becoming my own personal mantra.

The truth was, knowing what was coming next wouldn't do me much good anyway. Would it do much good for any of us? Isn't it true that we often have no idea what is actually good for us? Reflecting on when things had gone wrong in my past, I realized our tendency, as people, is to react like toddlers when we don't get what we want, throwing our toys and having a tantrum, only to look back a year later and say, "Thank goodness I didn't get what I wanted." Life tends to work itself out, and when something we want doesn't come to fruition, we frequently uncover a better opportunity later that sets us on the right path. So, there's no sense in getting too worked up over not getting what we want in life.

With that spark of insight, I decided to add to my new mantra: *We don't know what's good for us. Have security in the unknown.*

Weeks went by with zero meaningful progress in my job hunt. I ended up exploring options other than Dubai, too, particularly opportunities in the United Kingdom. Finally, however, I realized that I'd gone about my new job search in all the wrong ways. Yes, I had made the bold move to resign from my former role in order to focus on finding my new path forward in life. Yes, I had spent my days doing the proper work on myself. Those were all good things. But at the same time, I'd made one mistake: I was seeking the same sort of job in other countries as I'd been working here in JoBurg. I needed to let go of that career and open myself to a new career path that felt healthy for me—one that would take me where I wanted to go, not only physically in terms of a new city or new country but also mentally and spiritually in terms of the experience I could have while working it.

I knew I wanted to travel and have meaningful experiences and, of course, make some money along the way. Focusing on that, I detached from any particular outcome and trusted myself to find what I *really* needed next. Soon after that, I discovered exactly what that was—and it surprised the hell out of me.

The simplest conversation is what provided the spark of inspiration. Dave and I were talking things through one day, as we often did, when he casually mentioned a mutual friend of ours who had just made a career change of his own. He'd left a high-paying corporate job to go work on yachts as a deckhand with a longer-term goal of eventually becoming a yacht captain. After taking some courses, he was able to find work overseas.

I felt a pull in my chest and reached out to this person to learn more. Granted, I'd never worked on a boat. Sure, I'd grown up water skiing and wakeboarding and the like, and my dad raced rubber ducks[6], but I had no experience on anything like a yacht.

This mutual friend told me that the work could be fun and certainly had its perks, but there was a whole other side to it that was not

6 Small, fast speedboats built on aerodynamic rubber pontoons.

easy at all. Finding a position could be difficult—there were far more aspiring deckhands in the world than there were jobs for deckhands—and the work could be challenging. In fact, many aspiring deckhands left their lives behind to start over in new countries only to find themselves out of money and nearly homeless.

So, he recommended that, after taking the proper training courses, I move to the South of France, one of the best locations for a new deckhand to find day work and build a résumé. If I was going to have a real shot at making it in this industry, that was where I needed to be. Even still, he made clear that there were no guarantees in this world. You could do everything right to prepare for a career in yachting and still not find enough work to make a living.

As we spoke, however, such negative possibilities didn't concern me, and I felt more drawn toward the positives that this path could offer if things *did* work out: an average base salary of around 3,500 to 4,500 U.S. dollars, zero expenses while working on the yacht, and the opportunity to travel broadly along the way. I could earn money abroad in a strong foreign currency while seeing more of the world.

After some consideration, I decided to commit to this course. More than any money I could make, what appealed to me most was the experience that this offered. Something in me felt certain that by pursuing this, I would grow in ways that I needed—even if I couldn't see exactly what they were yet.

I had no idea just how true that would end up being.

I approached this new path the same way I do anything else: by diving in headfirst. To get started, I needed to spend a few weeks taking yachting courses that were available only in Cape Town, so I'd have to fly and stay there for a little while. After that, I planned to return to JoBurg for about a week, then fly to the South of France where I would begin looking for day work with a goal of eventually securing a full-time contract with a yacht crew. In the meantime, I would need to ensure that I had a few weeks' worth of living expenses in the bank to support myself while I sought a job.

Of course, money would be the biggest challenge. As a South African, at the time, the rand/euro exchange rate was at almost seventeen rand to one euro, meaning that everything I needed to do to make this a reality would cost me seventeen times more than someone else earning foreign currency. For starters, I needed living expenses saved for Cape Town *and* the South of France. In addition, to apply for a French visa, I had to show the government that I had purchased plane tickets into the country *and* out of the country, show proof of accommodations that had been paid up front, and prove I had a certain amount of money in my bank account. If I didn't have at least 5,000 euros saved, they wouldn't accept me into their country. That worked out to some 75,000 rand.

I understood the logic. They didn't want me running out of money and getting stranded, unable to leave France, because then I would become their problem. Still, this was going to be much more expensive than I'd anticipated.

Before leaving for Cape Town to start my yachting courses, I had to sell everything that I owned. I sold my motorbike, my BMW, and all my other possessions, and Dave even agreed to sell the house we had bought together. Since the money from the sale of the house would take some time to come through, I still found myself a bit short on cash. Fortunately, my uncle provided me "sponsorship" with my visa application by giving me a copy of his bank statements as surety that someone was able to get me back home if needed.

In addition, I had arranged with Glen to lend me some money to actually get my courses started, so everything seemed to be falling into place somewhat. However, when Dave was taking me to the airport to get from Johannesburg to Cape Town to begin my courses, I learned that the arrangement with Glen had fallen through. That meant I wouldn't have the money to actually pay for the courses once

I arrived at the school in Cape Town. For a moment, it appeared that my new journey had come to an abrupt halt, and the timing could not have been worse. Fortunately, like many times in my life, Dave pulled through for me without hesitation. He told me that he would front me the money, and when the house transfer went through, we would just settle then.

You know how, sometimes, when you want to do something, roadblocks seem to appear out of nowhere at every turn? In this situation, I was experiencing the opposite. As soon as I let go of needing to find a job I was familiar with, the yachting career presented itself. The moment I decided to commit to that, I was able to sell everything quickly, register for my courses, and secure my visa. With the help and support of amazing family and friends, I was able to overcome the little speed bumps along the way. Everything was falling into place, and every step of the way, I felt calm and confident that I was doing exactly what I needed to be doing next. I held my mantra in my mind: *Find security in the unknown.*

In Cape Town, things continued in kind. Meeting new people interested in the same line of work, staying in a hostel with some of those individuals, and even partying a bit with them made me feel like a new person in some ways. Since I was twenty-seven years old at this point, many of these people were younger than me, and being around their energy felt invigorating. So, too, did the fact that I was following the path I'd selected for myself, leaving my corporate career behind and setting off in pursuit of something that felt truly meaningful to me in ways that went beyond the security of a job or steady paycheck.

My courses went well, too, as we obtained our private watercraft licenses for jet skis and powerboats and learned basic safety training, life raft deployment, CPR, security, and anything else you can possibly think of that might have to do with working aboard a massive yacht.

Despite the uncertainty I knew awaited, I continued feeling tranquil. In addition to residing in a new city, surrounding myself with new people, and walking a rewarding new path, I was learning a new trade and acquiring skills and knowledge that would take me into the next stage of my life. For the first time, I felt that I had truly chosen the life I was living. I began to feel lighter, as though I had set down a burden I'd unknowingly been carrying. Nothing weighed me down anymore.

Upon completing my courses and returning to JoBurg, I finished selling my things and getting the rest of my affairs in order, then said my goodbyes. On a chilly autumn day, Dave, my mom, my stepdad, and my little brother took me to the airport to see me off to the South of France. As we shared some exciting and emotional farewell embraces, we all sort of felt like I might be a little crazy. I could tell that they still didn't really understand what was going on and what I was choosing to do with my life, but they were still being super supportive. My mom and stepdad had everyone join arms, and they recited a prayer of protection and safety over me as I entered my new adventure.

Then, in one of the most surreal moments of my life, I walked through the airport carrying everything I had left to my name in a single, carry-on-sized rolling suitcase.

The metaphor rang true to me in a powerful way: Maybe life is less about what we take with us and more about what we choose to leave behind. After all, when we are moving forward in life, we *have to* leave some things behind. That's how we make room for all that waits for us next.

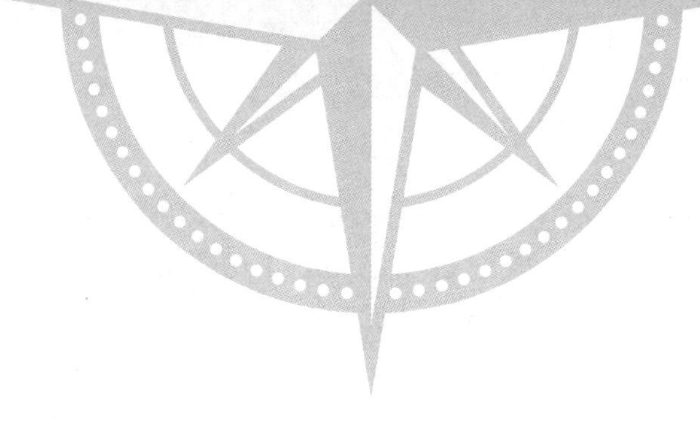

# CHAPTER 8

From the moment I arrived in the South of France, I felt the best kind of sensory overload. With no experience traveling internationally, I had to go through customs for the first time in my life and navigate public transportation from the airport to the place where I'd be staying. All the while, I was acutely aware I was in a new country where most of the people spoke French, a language I'd barely heard before. All of that stimulation I'd once craved and sought out in partying back in JoBurg I now experienced in full as I acclimated to my new surroundings. No night of dancing or partying compared to this. *This* was simply electrifying.

On the way through customs, part of me kept waiting for something to go awry. Maybe I had some paperwork wrong, or perhaps my visa wasn't processed properly. But no—everything worked out without a hitch.

Then, after making it out of the airport, I got a bit lost while trying to find the train station and ended up on a fifteen-minute hike outside of the airport. A few times, I had to stop and find someone who spoke English to ask for directions before eventually coming upon a tiny station. Realizing I must have missed the bigger station in the airport, I decided to just go for it with this one. It was all part of the adventure.

On the train ride toward the neighborhood of Antibes, where I would be staying in a yacht crew house, I took in the view through the train window and felt joy and excitement swelling in my chest as I caught a first glimpse the ocean. After making it to my stop, I emerged from the station in Antibes to see a marina and docks straight ahead of me. Taking a minute to appreciate the view, I breathed deeply, enjoying the heavy scent of saltwater, and felt a thrill at the fact that I was really doing this.

Another ten-minute walk later, I'd arrived at my new home on Av. Saint-Roch: a yellowish building with a bright red door. This was a yacht crew house where groups of yachties of all ages and levels of experience would bunk together while looking for their next job. Inside, the bottom floor of the house featured a kitchen, lounge, and basic amenities, while the second floor contained everybody's rooms. All of the furniture looked clean and modern and simple with a bamboo and wood aesthetic throughout. I would share a room with a few other people, all of us sleeping in bunk beds hostel style. Since we had a door leading to a small porch with a banister, we also had a clear view of the street below.

Throughout this initial process of getting into the country and reaching the crew house, I kept consciously checking in with myself in giddy excitement. *This is really what you're doing. You're in another country now. You've done everything that you had to do to get here, and you're starting another life now.* The fact that this really *was* my life felt beyond surreal, like taking your dream car for a drive only to be told that, no, this isn't just a joyride—this is your car now.

Upon arrival, some familiar faces greeted me as I recognized some of my mates who had taken the courses with me in Cape Town. We chatted and got to know the others staying at the crew house, some of whom got us up to speed on various details and dos and don'ts about the area and culture. The main thing seemed to be using common sense while socializing. This area had plenty of bars where scores of people in the yachting community liked to unwind, but none of them wanted to be harassed by greenies fresh off the train begging for work. Likewise, we were told: "Don't go out and become a sloppy, rowdy drunk. Socialize, have some fun, stay focused on your goals, respect people, put in the work, and, like everyone else, hope for the best."

After settling in a bit, my mind quickly turned to the small matter of actually finding work. Placement agencies existed in the yachting industry, and they could help me land jobs, but as long as I lacked true experience, they could do little to find me a contracted staff position on a boat. The first thing I needed to do was go down to the docks and do some day work, finding a crew that needed an extra hand for a day or two while their boat was in port. This sort of work would pay 150 euros or so per day and provide valuable experience and references for my résumé.

Of course, finding such day work is much easier said than done. Thousands of others just like me were in the South of France looking for their first boat gigs too. Competition would be fierce. Fortunately, that fit my competitive nature quite well, and with the lessons I'd learned about how much control I truly had over myself and my life, I felt self-assured, energized, and excited to take on this next challenge. I was secure in this next phase of the unknown.

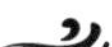

As my first order of business, I found a shop to print dozens of copies of my CV. The next morning, I woke up at 6 a.m.; put on my best boat shoes, chinos, belt, and white collared shirt; and took a train to one of the nearby docks in Monaco, stack of CVs in hand. I then spent the entire day walking the docks in every direction, introducing myself to various crew members I came across, handing out my CV to anybody who would take it, and asking everyone I met if they needed a day worker.

In this manner, I walked the docks until the sun set. By the end of the day, I was exhausted, out of résumés, and still jobless.

That night, I returned to the copy shop and printed off a fresh batch of résumés. Then, the following morning, I went to another dock.

Same story that day.

And the day after that.

And the day after that.

And the day after that.

This went on for one week . . . then two . . . then three. For three full weeks, I walked the docks from Cannes to Monaco and found no work. Everywhere I went, I was just one hopeful day worker in a sea of them, and there were far more of us than there were jobs.

I sure hoped I'd find that work soon though. After three weeks of this, I was running out of money. Rent at the crew house cost about 180 euros per week. Then, there was the cost of food, printing copies of my résumé, other necessities, and going out with my new friends. The South of France was much more expensive than Johannesburg, and since the rand is nearly twenty times weaker than the euro, I was hemorrhaging cash.

In the crew house, as I became friendly with people, an interesting dynamic unfolded: We all shared a common quest to make a living doing this work, which made us want to root for each other—and yet, at the same time, we were in competition with each other for that work. People returned to the crew house every night announcing their first day work gig or, better yet, their first contract, and we always made sure to celebrate with them for that. But while I was struggling to find work myself, I sometimes found myself becoming jealous.

When I sensed that negative emotion beginning to rise in me, I reminded myself of what I'd learned about my subconscious and consciously told myself to hold onto a mindset of celebration for my new friends. I truly believed things were still going to work out for me and held fast to my faith in the path I was walking. When someone else landed a new gig, I thought, *Good for them!* My time hadn't come yet, but I knew that failure was not an option at this point, and I never lost hope. The right job would arrive at the right time.

After all, I was now living through just how hard it was to get these gigs—and every gig somebody else got gave me proof that I could attain that work too.

~

One evening at Port Juan-les-Pins, weary after yet another long and fruitless day of walking the docks, I saw a navy-blue hull with the name *The Gene Machine.* Paired with that was a unique emblem: four symbols that reminded me of the PlayStation controller buttons. Something about this boat just seemed different. The crew had gathered on the back of the boat, seemingly engaged in their end-of-day meeting. When I caught the eye of one of them, I waved. He responded immediately and waved back vigorously, gesturing for me to approach.

"Hey, you!" he shouted in a thick French accent. "You are looking for work, yeah?"

*Yes, I'm looking for work!* was my emphatic mental reply.

Externally, I calmly replied, "Why yes, as a matter of fact, I am."

The man met me at the edge of the boat, asked for my CV, and looked it over while I tried to maintain my composure. This guy with a French accent who was on a super cool-looking boat was actually giving me the time of day after I'd spent weeks trying to find work. I felt like a guy in a movie trying to talk to a girl who's always been his biggest crush.

"Okay," the Frenchman finally said. "Be here tomorrow—7:30 a.m."

*Hell yes! You just gave me my first bit of day work!* I screamed on the inside.

But I maintained my cool, professional demeanor. "Sounds good. Thank you! See you tomorrow."

~

As it turned out, *The Gene Machine* was a well-known—and totally badass—exploration yacht. For one thing, it carried virtually every sort of watercraft toy you could imagine. For another, it was equipped to go almost anywhere in the world at a moment's notice. In short, *The Gene Machine* was one of the most recognizable yachts in the South of France, and a spot on its crew was one of the most coveted opportunities. This was one of the best day work gigs I could have for my résumé.

As a day worker, I was doing all the dirty work that the crew didn't necessarily want to do—scrubbing teak, doing a massive top-to-bottom washdown of the entire boat, and performing other tasks of that nature. The crew and I got along well, however, and I felt their appreciation for the work I was doing. The Frenchman turned out to be the yacht's bosun[7], and he had one of the best, most down-to-earth leadership styles a crew could want.

I went about my work with the same mentality I had once gone about sports and, later, my dance performances. Even though I no longer had an audience, I worked as though somebody was always watching me. No cutting corners, always doing a bit extra wherever I could find extra to do, and not feeling finished with a task until I could think of nothing else that could possibly be done to improve on the situation. My mindset was simple and straightforward: I am going to do this work properly.

As I worked, I dropped several not-so-subtle hints about my interest in joining the crew on a full contract. That was my ultimate goal here, after all. Unfortunately, they had a full crew and didn't need any new members. Even still, one day's work turned into three days, earning me 450 euros that would secure my bunk in the crew house for few more weeks. I also received a brilliant reference letter and a valuable bit of experience to add to my résumé. To further boost my spirits, as I departed the boat, the Frenchman assured me that as soon as they needed another full-time crew member, I would get the call.

One week later, I landed a five-day gig working a much bigger boat, which put another 800 euros in my pocket. Just like that, I was

7 A bosun leads the deck crew of a yacht.

squared away for two full months and had two excellent jobs on my CV. That was how quickly things turned around. Now that I had some money and was sensing momentum on my side, I began to enjoy myself a bit more as well, going out on weekends to drink with my new friends and network with others in the yachting community.

Again, I found myself marveling at the life I was living and thinking about how much control I truly had over my circumstances as long as I maintained the proper mindset. With all this in mind, I couldn't help feeling overwhelmingly grateful for all that I'd learned that had brought me here. All I needed to do now was keep finding day work until a proper full-time crew opportunity came along. In my mind, nothing could stop me.

Little did I know, life was about to take one hell of a nosedive.

One night, while I slept peacefully in the crew house, the fairytale life I was living suddenly turned into a nightmare. I awoke to flashlights in my face, pointed at me by men wielding automatic weapons.

*Oh, shit. Now what?*

# CHAPTER 9

An hour later, I was sitting in a police station with my bunkmates, all of us asking each other the same question: *What the hell is going on?*

All we knew was that the police had raided our crew house, taken all our passports, loaded us into cars, and brought us here. They all spoke French, none of them spoke English, and we spent the rest of the day at the station simply waiting for a translator.

When the translator arrived, we learned that one of the newest residents of the crew house had been found unconscious in the street outside of our building around 3 a.m. He was suffering from severe wounds to his body and head as the victim of an apparent attack. Now, he was in a coma in the hospital where doctors didn't know whether he would survive. His parents had flown in, distressed, irate, and intent on justice. We were all suspects.

Working with the translator, the police took each of our statements individually. After holding us at the station for a day and a half, they finally allowed us to return to the crew house, but they instructed us to not leave port, and they kept our passports. We couldn't leave the country until the case was closed. The idea that we could end up in prison for a crime we didn't commit stayed at the forefront of our minds, leaving us terrified. To top it all off, I'd finally worked so hard to put myself in a position to get my dream yacht job—but now, if somebody called to offer me a contract with a crew, I couldn't even go.

We lived like this for about two weeks.

And then, just as suddenly as the situated arose, it resolved. The man who'd initially called an ambulance, a taxicab driver, gave a statement testifying that he had seen the victim go to the balcony of his room, urinate over the edge of the banister, and fall. After dropping one and a half stories down, the man hit a car, bounced off, and crumpled on the pavement. What the police had been trying to sort out was whether the man had been pushed over the edge of the banister or had simply fallen over on his own.

Well, the victim had a friend who'd traveled to France with him, and that friend told the police that this sort of thing had happened before. Evidently, the victim had a pattern of going out, getting too drunk, and finding unconventional locations in which to relieve himself. Without any evidence that the victim had been pushed and without any motive found for anybody to push him, the police concluded that it was all an unfortunate accident. Nobody would be charged, the case was closed, and the police returned our passports. I was free again.

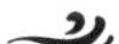

For a couple of months after that, as if the universe were rewarding me for the fright with the police, I found a steady stream of day work. This took me aboard different boats in the ports and further taught me how various crews worked together, giving me a bigger itch than ever to join a crew full time myself.

But then, as suddenly as all that work had come in, it dried up again. I went a full month without landing a single day work gig, and once again, I began to run out of money. In time, at the end of my days walking the docks, I found myself watching the waves roll in and listening to them slowly *clap, clap, clap* against the side of the docks. I'd just sit there and reflect.

For a couple of months, I'd felt as though I had this world somewhat figured out. As though I'd started to find my place in it with my regular day work. As though I belonged here and a full-time contract with a crew was inevitable. Now, I'd begun to feel uncomfortable—out of place.

I wasn't alone. One of my crew house mates, Jason, started feeling the same way. The number of jobs available here simply didn't align with the much larger number of yachties looking for work. We discussed options, such as moving to Italy with a few others from the crew house; the cost of living was lower, and we could share a place and just walk the docks there. Or we could go to Spain, where a major yacht hub would surely offer more jobs.

None of those plans quite moved along, however, and one night, sitting in my bunk and looking at my bank account, I thought I might really be reaching the end of my journey. All I had left to my name was fifty euros.

This should have filled me with desperation or fear, and sure, I felt a bit confused and uncertain of what was coming next. But to my pleasant surprise, I found myself experiencing the same calm confidence I'd felt all along. Part of me even found the situation amusing because, on one hand, I imagined what it would be like to go home with my tail tucked between my legs, appearing to have somewhat failed at this whole endeavor. On the other hand, I didn't even know how I would *get* home. The plane ticket home that the French government had required me to purchase had expired, and now I didn't have enough money for a new ticket.

Knowing I faced a dire situation, I remained self-assured, holding true to the lessons I had learned and was determined to live by. I kept myself in the mindset of what I wanted to happen, not what I was afraid might happen. I remained light in my nature, even as I continued hustling day after day on the docks while my bank account dwindled. Naturally, I felt the stress of knowing that *something* needed to happen in order for me to get work and make money again, but

I recognized the value in not allowing myself to slip into a heavy or stressful mentality. All that would do was deplete my energy and rob me of the joy still to be found in the moment.

*Besides*, I reminded myself, *I still have fifty euros.*

Against all logic, I felt in my bones that this was not the end—failure was not an option for me here. I didn't know what was going to happen, but I knew that *something* would—soon—and it was going to be good. I felt so certain that I decided to go out that night and have some drinks rather than just stay holed up in the crew house. Maybe I didn't know what the future held, but in that moment, I knew that I wanted to be around people. So, I gathered some of my mates, and we went to a bar.

Specifically, we went to the Hop Store, a favorite spot for yachties in the South of France. I couldn't afford to be there—my beer cost five euros. I'd just put 10 percent of my net worth toward a pint. Choosing to remain light about it, I finished my drink and had another, consciously having fun conversations, enjoying the music, and staying in the moment. All my challenges aside, I was still drinking in a bar in the South of France, surrounded by people who loved the same work I loved, all of us trying to make it in a challenging industry, simultaneously competing with each other and in it together. That was all I needed to focus on.

Over the course of the night, I heard a familiar English accent, and next thing I knew, I was talking with the lead deckhand of *The Gene Machine,* the first boat on which I'd done day work. After some chitchat, he told me that they were preparing for a massive trip.

Now, most people who own luxury superyachts do what we call "milk runs"—simple outings between Italy and France, mostly staying within the Mediterranean. *The Gene Machine,* however, was an expedition yacht, and its owner had a seventy-five-day itinerary planned for their upcoming trip. They would leave the South of France, arc around Europe, all the way up past Norway, and move into Svalbard, Norway's northernmost island. From there, they'd go beyond Greenland and proceed as far north and as deep into the pack ice as they could go.

Their goal was to break the record for going farther north than any luxury superyacht had ever gone. A full-blown Arctic expedition, this was going to be an epic, once-in-a-lifetime opportunity for a yacht crew. An absolute dream job.

"So," I asked, "do you need another crew member?"

He laughed and said no, they had a full crew—but they did need a day worker for a few days to prepare for the journey. The gig was mine if I wanted it.

Just like that, I had work lined up to cover my rent in France for another month.

That night, I could have stayed in my bunk, hoping to find day work the next time I went walking the docks. Instead, I'd gone with my gut when I wanted to be around people and enjoy myself. In trusting my intuition, I'd now found some more work—and I'd found it by doing what I loved most: just hanging out with cool people in a bar.

To celebrate, I spent half of what was left in my bank account on tequilas.

Upon arrival to the boat, my excitement at the new gig quickly leveled out, and my heart dropped as I realized something: the crew had a new junior deckhand for their upcoming Arctic expedition. *What the hell?* was all I could think at first. As grateful as I was for the day work, in my mind, they should have asked me to join the full-time crew first—like they'd said they would.

There would be no complaining or moping, however. My competitive instincts kicked in, and I decided that I would show the crew that they had made a terrible mistake. For the next few days, I would work my ass off and make a massive impression on the members of *The Gene Machine* crew.

After spending the first day and a half or so performing more menial tasks, we got to work on giving *The Gene Machine* a full washdown.

Here, I went into sixth gear after being given the assignment to scrub the teak. To do this, we used something called *oxalic acid* that leaves burns and blisters if you let it get on your skin. Although we wore rubber gloves and boots as protection, inevitably, some of the acid would find its way onto my skin. In addition, the boots chafed, leaving the flesh on my shins and my knees vulnerable to one terribly painful situation.

Nevertheless, I refused to stop working, telling myself that the wounds would heal and any pain I felt would be worth the impression I'd leave on that crew. Working the port side of the boat, I scrubbed the bloody hell out of the teak on the deck and ensured that not a single inch went untouched. Although nobody was watching me work, I maintained that mentality as usual, knowing that I wanted to leave this job with zero doubt that I had given my duties my all. For their next expedition, I wanted to be the first call this crew made when they needed a new Member.

After all the scrubbing—and the bleeding—my frustration remained, but my work was done. The crew invited me to the aft deck for a beer at sunset. In that moment, I found perspective, and the frustration finally faded. Drinking a beer aboard a luxury superyacht will have that effect. Yes, I wished I'd been chosen for this expedition with this crew. Even still, they paid me well, I did good work, I made a good impression, and my life continued apace in the direction of my dreams.

Upon finishing my beer, the yacht's chief officer summoned me to the wheelhouse. Paycheck time. When I reached the wheelhouse, I found not only the chief officer waiting for me but the captain as well.

The captain asked me how things had gone during my time aboard his ship and how I'd enjoyed the work. I told him things had gone great. In fact, I believe I said, "Flippin' awesome." Plus, I told him that I loved working with his crew and enjoyed doing the work itself. Bloody shins and all. Then, I made my soft but clear pitch, telling him that if he ever had an opening on his crew again someday, I'd love to be considered for a full-time position.

With that, the chief officer offered the envelope containing my money, and I reached out to take it from him—but he wouldn't let it go.

"So," he said, "you can take this and go—or I can keep this and, instead, give you this . . . " With his other hand, he presented a piece of paper. "We would like to offer you a job on the boat right now," the chief officer went on, "for *this* trip."

The piece of paper contained the terms of a contract awaiting my signature.

Of course, I signed immediately. I listened in near disbelief as they explained their decision. They had developed concerns over the new crew member's capacity to manage the extreme conditions and many unexpected challenges inherent to a seventy-five-day Arctic expedition. They had been questioning their decision to hire that person for the past few days, and on our last day of work, they chose to offer the job to me instead.

One thing in particular finally pushed them over the edge. They took me to the balcony of the wheelhouse that overlooked the bow of the ship, then told me to look at the deck and tell them what I saw. One side of the deck appeared to be a slightly brighter shade of color than the other. Unbeknownst to me, as I'd cleaned the port side of the yacht, the new crew member had been assigned the starboard side. Although the captain and chief officer hadn't intended for this to be some sort of competition for the job, that's effectively what it became. While they stood right here, deliberating over the new crew member, they glanced across the ship, noticed the different quality of work, and realized they had their answer. My side shined brighter.

Even when you think nobody's watching you, do things as though somebody *is* watching you—because one day, they just might be.

After the best commute of my life, back at the crew house, we celebrated. Finally, I had become the person celebrating their amazing new job instead of just the person waiting for the new job to arrive. That night, we partied.

The next morning, as I traveled back to *The Gene Machine* with my packed bags and months of adventure ahead, I basked in the significance of this moment. All the seemingly impulsive decisions I had made, all that I had discovered about my subconscious mind, all the lessons I had learned and my efforts to live according to those lessons—everything had all worked out.

As I stepped aboard *The Gene Machine* and joined my new crew, I recognized I was starting the dream job I had come all this way to find. More than that, I was arriving at the moment I had long believed to be possible for me, even when I'd had no good reason to maintain my faith. The journey to this point had rendered many challenging moments, bouts of exhaustion, and more than enough heartache and pain. But I had made it. Wounds heal, and the scars our wounds leave behind remind us of how strong we can be.

To this day, I still have acid burn scars on my legs.

# CHAPTER 10

Before leaving port to pick up the yacht owners in Monaco, we did a couple of days' worth of work in preparation for the expedition. The covers came off couches and floors, and we polished all the newly exposed areas. We also pulled out all the toys and made sure they were fueled, oiled, and otherwise in proper working order. Plus, the bosun helped familiarize me with various moving parts of the job. He shared tips for correct line handling and what to look out for when leaving port.

While I worked, the significance of this new experience stayed forefront in my mind. I felt as though I had truly reached a new level in my life, and I was determined to soak up every tiny part of the experience. Each stage of your life requires a different version of yourself, and I was looking forward to meeting who I would become next.

For starters, as the new man on crew in my first job in the industry, I knew that meant starting at the bottom of the pecking order. This was a bit of an adjustment because I was older than some of my superiors. After having worked my way up in corporate and entertainment jobs to achieve a bit of status and even manage people back home, now I was the low man on the totem pole again. That would mean taking on the dirty work—being one of the first people awake every morning to wipe the dew off the boat, polish the stainless steel railings, etc.; setting up the toys; blowing up the inflatables for the kids every morning and packing them away at the end of the day; rinsing and shammying the deck in every port; and all manner of other tasks. Many nights while in port, that also meant taking on passerelle duty when the guests went off boat, meaning I had to stay awake on deck while the rest of the crew went to sleep, ensuring that nobody trespassed onboard and greeting the guests upon their return.

This was a humbling position for me but in a wonderful way. My role was to listen to orders and dutifully complete the tasks I'd been instructed to do. I saw this as my newest challenge, and I embraced it. Growing up playing sports, I understood the importance of everyone on a team knowing their role and owning it. In this situation, as the new man on the team, that meant simply saying "Yes, sir" and "Thank you, sir" to my superiors and giving them respect, no matter what they asked of me. No amount of talking or discussion would accomplish as much as—in a sense—simply letting my game do my talking for me. In this case, that involved keeping my head down and continuing to do my work as well as I'd done it to earn the job in the first place. Having played years of rugby growing up, I found myself also drawing on lessons of commitment, discipline, and focus.

This crew made such things easier, too, as they fostered a good and healthy work environment from the outset. The captain, chief officer, and bosun alike all managed the ship in a positive manner. While the captain ran a tight ship and commanded respect, he also treated the crew with respect in return. I found his leadership abilities impressive since, at twenty-nine years old, he was also rather young. He made us feel comfortable, and he seemed cool and approachable but also gave us a clear sense that we should not step out of line.

In addition, I'd never been out to sea aboard a yacht this size before, let alone a yacht so fully equipped. At fifty-five meters in length, *The Gene Machine* contained everything we could possibly need for our Arctic expedition. Plus, the boat carried every water toy you could imagine, including Jetsurfs, jet skis, wakeboards, kneeboards, kitesurfing gear, and even a sailboat. As for the yacht and the expedition itself, I quickly realized just how much I had to learn about tasks such as operating lines and fenders, identifying and announcing landmarks to the captain, and all manner of expedition yacht duties.

Was this a tremendous challenge? Of course. But the challenges I faced only deepened my satisfaction with this new phase in my life.

After finishing our prep work, to share a final meal before departure, the entire crew went to Nikki Beach in Cannes, a well-known hotspot right on the beach with sweeping views of the ocean. Growing up in South Africa, I frequently heard people talk about traveling to Europe, and Nikki Beach always came up in those conversations as one place you just had to go.

As we drank champagne and ate sushi, the significance of this moment continued to swell, and a wave of emotion rolled over me once again. Not only had I made it to the South of France and earned a contract for an expedition—I was also now a member of a crew.

*I really made it*, I thought.

Being on this crew gave me a deep sense of belonging that felt almost tribal. It was something I had craved all my life. As I mentioned previously, coming from a divorced home, I'd never truly felt like I belonged to a family. Of course, I loved my parents and was extremely close with Jacques and Uncle Kosie and their family. Plus, I experienced a sense of kinship with my teammates while playing sports as I grew up. And none of this is to discount the other friends I had, too, who all meant a great deal to me. But while I still trained regularly to remain fit and healthy, team sports had run their course in my life, and as time had gone on, my various relationships had, for one reason or another, shifted and faded in various ways.

So far in the South of France, although I'd developed some camaraderie with people I'd met in the bunk house and at bars, my quest to land consistent yachting work had been essentially a solo venture with plenty of lonely moments. Aboard *The Gene Machine,* however, as a member of this crew, I discovered that sense of unity I'd been longing to find. Working together, eating together, drinking together, we quickly came to feel a genuine sense of care for each other. Knowing what we were on the precipice of encountering deepened our immediate bond. We were about to spend two and a half months at sea with a goal of venturing as far north as a luxury superyacht had ever gone. Whatever the sea had waiting for us, we would face it together.

The next morning, as we pulled out of port the first time, I was captivated by the magnitude of our boat in contrast to the narrow confines of the marina. As the bow started to move, I felt a surge of adrenaline and anxiety as we navigated through the docks and past all the other watercraft. This was quite a tight space, we were an enormous yacht, and the severity of a potential mistake really struck me. All of us had to be on our game, listening to callsigns from the captain as we manned the fenders in various locations and ensured that we exited the harbor free of damage.

Once we'd cleared the channel, I felt a sense of relief while I finished packing away the lines and securing the fenders. As we entered the open ocean, I turned to look back whence we came—and was stunned by the breathtaking view. Walking to the bow of the yacht, I soaked in the view as the South of France began to fade into the horizon. After having spent the last few months there on land, to see the region from this perspective gave me a new appreciation for its beauty. Under the rising sun, the land that had once seemed like a gigantic, far-off dream now began to shrink behind us as the open sea beckoned ahead.

My radio crackled, and then the captain spoke to me: "It's beautiful, right?"

I turned to see him watching me from his perch in the wheelhouse. He had a big grin on his face, and when he laughed, I laughed back. That meant a lot to me. The captain had just reached out to me, a brand-new junior deckhand and the lowest member of his crew, and acknowledged the moment I was having.

As I returned my gaze to the sea, a flood of emotion washed over me. Every mile we were about to travel was a mile I'd never traveled before. I deeply felt the weight of this moment—a profound sense of awe, gratitude, and anticipation for the journey that lay ahead, both aboard *The Gene Machine* and in the next phase of my life.

Cruising the smooth, blue-green waters of the Mediterranean Sea, we were pleased to find our initial leg of the trip gave us an easy, glamorous start to the voyage. First, we stopped in Monaco to pick up the yacht owner and his family: a wealthy geneticist and inventor and his wife and three children. They were fantastic owners—warm and friendly. With sincere benevolence, they invited us to participate with them in their various activities and to use their watersport toys as our own when we had free time. Even though I was new to the industry, I knew that such generosity wasn't always common and felt humbled and grateful to begin my yachting experience with such excellent guests.

As we made our way through the Mediterranean, I found myself thinking of my father. When we anchored in Monaco, as we sat in the harbor within walking distance of the Formula 1 Grand Prix route, I reflected on his passion for F1 racing—a passion shared by most sports fans in South Africa. The Monaco race each year was the one we most anticipated, and he always spoke about how amazing it would be to actually go and watch the Monaco Grand Prix. Well, I got to do this during my time in France. I actually walked on the very track that my dad and I dreamed about together. Life was totally surreal to me during moments like this.

After Monaco, we made stops in places such as Spain and Ibiza. While at the latter, I remembered some of my father's stories about the parties and other fun that would happen there. We were too busy working to partake in the party scene, but we still had time to knock off for a nice meal and a beer together in the city. Working in shifts, some of us would go out to eat together while others remained aboard to keep watch over the ship. Even simply sitting there, drinking a beer with the crew and looking smart in our uniforms, gave me a wonderful experience to remember.

As our journey continued, I learned as much as I could about my new job, spending every day developing my abilities and acclimating to life spent round the clock on a yacht. Members of the crew introduced me to the intricacies of running a boat, and the bosun taught me various necessary skills I had no way to learn as a mere day worker.

I approached these new skills with the same rigor and discipline I'd once applied to learning karate and other sports—by doing countless repetitions of the same exercise. For instance, the bosun gave me a piece of line and showed me new knots to practice tying, so whenever the guests were off the boat and I had down time, I sat alone in my cabin with the line and tied knot after knot after knot until I felt confident in them.

In a pleasant surprise, however, some of those old skills also proved beneficial. No matter how much life might change, we always carry parts of ourselves onto our new paths, and that will help us in unexpected ways. In this case, my fitness training experience became appealing to the yacht owner and his family. In fact, they started requesting regular personal training sessions. Next thing I knew, I found myself on the deck of this luxury superyacht every morning, watching some of the most stunning sunrises I could have ever imagined, doing something I deeply loved while genuinely helping people—all as part of my new career.

To call this a dream come true seems insufficient. This felt like being in some sort of fantastical movie, living exactly the life I wanted, full of adventure and travel and beauty. And I was doing it on a fifty-five-million-dollar yacht, eating food prepared by chefs, working with an incredible crew, and challenging myself in the most awesome way. I was even being compensated for being here and didn't have to pay for so much as a toothbrush. In exchange, all I had to do was keep a boat clean and well-maintained and make other people feel safe, entertained, and happy. What more could I ask for?

Day after day, as I stood on the deck of the yacht and felt endless awe at my new life, I just kept thinking, *I am so freaking lucky.*

Soon thereafter, I realized just how lucky I truly was, as I made a mistake that nearly resulted in my being kicked off the boat.

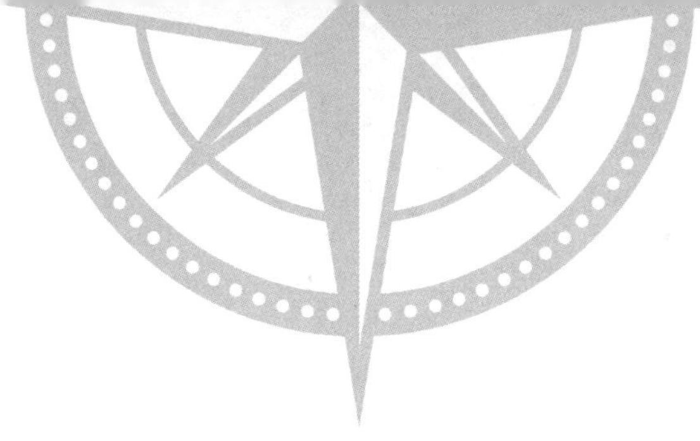

# CHAPTER 11

Making our way out of the Mediterranean and toward the United Kingdom, we traveled down the River Thames to our next big stop, London. From there, we made for Amsterdam. While there, I discovered—not for the first time or the last—that life always has a funny way of bringing you back down to earth and making sure you stay in line.

This began with a fun and wild night as I lived out an experience that only seemed to exist on television. The captain gave our crew a night of leave, along with strict orders to return to the docks by a certain time. To reach the docks from the yacht, we took the tender[8], and the captain said no more tender trips would be allowed past the given curfew.

Determined to make the most of our night, I spent half of my weekly salary as we drank and partied our way through the red-light district. The bosun assisted wholeheartedly in this seizing of the moment, having fast become a good friend as he turned out to be a fellow hooligan. Fun to be around and one excellent drinker, he enjoyed pushing limits as much as I did—and we pushed hard on this night.

Next thing we knew, curfew had come and gone, and by the time we reached the docks, the tender had been back at the yacht for a good two hours. The bosun, ever the problem-solver, quickly took

8 The thirty-foot motorboat that comes with the yacht.

action on a plan that, at the time, seemed genius and infallible. He dove into the water, swam to the yacht, commandeered said tender, and provided us water taxi service back to the ship. From our not-quite-sober perspective, we deemed this nothing more than harmless drunken shenanigans.

The next morning, we discovered that the captain didn't see things quite the same way. He called us to the wheelhouse, announced that he had reviewed the previous evening's security footage, and—well, let's just say that he expressed his displeasure in no uncertain terms.

First off, we'd been late, meaning that we had completely disrespected the captain's explicit orders.

Second, we'd been reckless to the point of dangerous. In the sober light of day, our shenanigans didn't seem quite so harmless. The bosun, completely intoxicated, had dove into cold waters in the dead of night, swum to the yacht, taken the tender and, in his state of inebriation, piloted it to the dock. At that point, he had picked up the rest of us, a group of hooligans equally inebriated. All of this with guests on board and under our care.

In addition, the next leg of our journey would require diligence and rigorous attention to detail as we approached complicated maneuvers, choppy seas, and, ultimately, the frigid, ice-packed, and potentially deadly waters of Svalbard and beyond. Everybody on board needed to be at the top of their game, and the choices we had made that night in Amsterdam had given the captain good cause for concern about our preparedness for what lay ahead. To be a good crew member, you not only needed to do your job and do it well, but you needed to comport yourself in a way that didn't create additional stress or doubt about your *ability* to do your job well. We'd behaved like children, and the captain could not rely on children.

"If any of you do anything like this again," the captain said, "you're off the boat."

This showed me that as good and glamorous as life could become, I needed to recognize just how quickly I could mess that up as well.

The lessons I'd learned from the TAG course and from Dr. DeMartini's talks came back to mind, specifically those regarding the way that life will always find a way to balance out if you fail to maintain balance within yourself. You need to know your boundaries and your limits and pay close attention to when you approach them. After all, you can be living out one of the best opportunities of your life and then destroy the entire situation in a single night if you're not careful.

Believe it or not, I found myself feeling appreciative that this had happened. This served as a wakeup call and a beneficial reminder of a valuable lesson. In one sense, I had put both my feet in one boat by committing to my dreams in the yachting industry. But internally, I still lived with one foot in the boat of professionalism, discipline, building a healthy bank account, and growing a good life for myself and the other foot in the boat of being a free spirit committed to always having an epic time.

I still had much to learn about life. More immediately, I also had much to learn about the sea itself and just how dangerous it could be.

Life once again providing balance, a moment of sheer beauty followed. After leaving Amsterdam, we continued pushing northward to Switzerland and Sweden, where we began moving inland through smaller rivers and lakes. As we approached Sweden's Lake Vänern, one of the biggest lakes in Europe, we first had to navigate the Trollhätte Canal.

Contact with the sides of the canal became inevitable due to the size of our yacht, so we deployed the fenders. Next, we set about navigating six different lochs that served as a yacht-sized staircase of water. Upon entering the first one, we docked for fifteen to twenty minutes, tying the yacht to the shore while the loch filled with water. Taking the role of man on the land, I disembarked to ensure the lines were secured, and then we waited for the loch to fill, elevating the yacht in this first loch to the level of the subsequent loch.

While waiting, I took in the view: gorgeous, lush green landscapes and spectacular blue skies. Not so long ago, I'd stood in an office urinal feeling like a man in jail. Now, here I was, being paid to work in picturesque Sweden.

When the loch finished filling, I untied the yacht to free it from its docking station, and the captain piloted the boat through the gates into the next loch while I ran alongside. We repeated this process until we'd reached the top of the lochs, where, upon entering Lake Vänern, we found ourselves greeted by a crowd that had gathered to witness this massive yacht passing through.

As we made our way across the lake, we dropped anchor to allow the guests to enjoy their jet skis and other water toys. Unfortunately, conditions took a rough and stormy turn. The water became as choppy as the deep ocean, and we needed to move to a new location. Two jet skis remained in the water, but docking them in the yacht proved more challenging than was worth the trouble, so the captain asked me and another crew member if we felt comfortable simply driving the jet skis behind the yacht as we moved.

I believe my reaction was something to the effect of: "Sweet!"

The captain warned us to exercise caution due to the rough conditions and to pace ourselves due to the lengthy distance we had to cover to reach our next location. But naturally, we let ourselves immediately get carried away. As the yacht set off and we fired up the jet skis, we quickly gave ourselves over to the impulse to drive them like we were Hollywood stuntmen. The massive waves weren't dangerous—they were gifts from the sea gods, aquatic ramps off of which to launch ourselves.

Well, our enthusiasm for such behavior lasted all of ten minutes, at which point we realized we were already exhausted. My arms and legs were throbbing and weak. The swells had risen to roughly ten feet high, conditions were intensifying, and we were losing ground on the yacht. Realizing that—surprise, surprise—the captain had been right, we stopped our shenanigans, sharpened our focus, and did our duty.

The waves made that as hard for us as they could. We found ourselves sent flying off swell after swell, going airborne on these jet skis—against our will now—and slamming back down into the water. *Ba-bow! Ba-bow! Ba-bow!*

As we crashed into wave after wave, we used all of our arm, leg, and core strength to support ourselves. After forty-five minutes of this, our muscles started to give way, and I wasn't having fun anymore. In a lifetime of riding jet skis, motorbikes, and the like, I'd never been this tired. We had no clear sense of how much further we had to go, and this had rapidly gone from fun adventure to challenging job task to a matter of survival.

Then came one especially gargantuan wave, followed by another from a different direction, followed by yet one more. *Ba-bow! Ba-bow! Ba-bow!* My arm gave out, and I fell straight down onto the front of the jet ski. My face hit first, smashing the handlebars and giving me a deep gash straight through my lip.

To my immense relief, we reached our new anchorage location shortly thereafter—but after docking the jet ski and returning to deck, the chief officer greeted me with, "What the bloody hell?"

The expression was quite literal. Blood was dripping down my face.

"Yep," I said. "Conditions were rough out there."

There I was, third week on the yacht, newest crew member, bottom of the totem pole, pissing blood all over the boat after busting my face open just driving a flippin' jet ski.

Thankfully, my lip didn't require stitches, and the incident became a running joke. Everyone watch out when Ashton gets near the jet skis!

This also gave me a healthier appreciation and respect for exactly what we could face on the yacht—not to mention, it taught me to take my job more seriously. Perhaps I had landed my dream job, and with it, I got to have some fun. However, I couldn't keep forgetting that this was serious work, too, and I needed to take care of myself so that I could stay on top of my responsibilities. I didn't want to add stress to the crew or create a negative experience for our guests.

Frankly, my behavior had been reckless on the jet ski. I could have easily hit my head instead of my lip. That could have knocked me unconscious and created an entirely different and more dangerous situation that would've threatened not only my life but also the lives of the crewmates who would have had to rescue me. The sea, especially in dicey conditions, always deserves respect.

This lesson left me with a nice, lasting memento too. I needed to take the photo for my UK passport a few days later, and there was my big, busted lip front and center.

Next up, we made passage for the highlight of the trip and our ultimate destination: Norway—and, beyond it, Svalbard and the ice. We were about to go farther than any luxury superyacht had ever gone.

# CHAPTER 12

After navigating through various rivers and tributaries, we came upon water as smooth as glass and bordered by mountains rising on both sides of us with waterfalls as far as the eye could see. We had reached the fjords of Norway. It felt like a magical, dreamlike place.

As part of our agenda for this location, the boss and his family wanted to paraglide from a mountain atop the fjords. Finding a proper location, the captain backed the yacht toward land, dropped anchor, created proper tension on the anchor line, and then sent us to swim two lines to shore, where we securely tied off the yacht.

Then, the boss invited me to go paragliding with him and his family. They had always been great about keeping all of us on the crew involved in their activities, wanting to create and maintain good, fun vibes throughout the excursion. We all felt grateful for that, knowing that many yacht owners treat the crew like second-class citizens simply there to do a job. This guy was awesome, thoughtfully rotating through crew members to join them on each activity.

After disembarking, we took a car partway up one of the fjords and then reached a point where we had to continue on foot, hiking to the peak. Upon reaching the summit, we strapped into our parachute and leapt, soaring over the fjords as we glided above the yacht and landed in a nearby field.

The sheer magnificence of this experience overwhelmed me. I can safely say this was one of the most breathtaking moments of my life. Standing atop this mountain, looking out at the glassy waters below and the verdant mountains rising all around, I felt almost dizzy with appreciation of how, once again, I found myself so far from where I once was in every way—physically, emotionally, psychologically, even spiritually.

That corporate job I'd once been so afraid of leaving now felt like a distant memory. I'd taken that leap into the unknown and trusted myself to find a way forward. I'd stayed true to myself, sold all my possessions, and endured one challenge after another, knowing where I wanted to go but not sure how I could get there. Just a few weeks prior, I'd been down to my last fifty euros. Now, I was *here,* flying through the fjords of Norway, one of the most beautiful places on earth.

Every new stage of this expedition also felt like entering a new stage of my life and of my personal development, and the indescribably gorgeous surroundings I continued to encounter aligned beautifully with that.

After all, your outer world reflects your inner world.

As we continued through Norway, we spent some time in various cities and small towns interacting with the locals. Not only did Norway have fantastic landscapes, but the country also contained incredible people. Some places you visit on this planet just feel more special than others. Norway is one of those places.

At some point throughout our voyage, I made an offhand comment to another member of the crew that if we had some cameras and producers aboard, everything we were doing would make for one hell of a reality television show. I didn't think people would believe everything that happened on these superyachts and all the work it took to make it happen.

He laughed and told me a show like that already existed—*Below Deck*. I'd never heard of it. They didn't go on full expeditions like we did, but they'd spend a few days out at sea. The show would center around all that went on aboard a yacht for the guests as well as how crew members from all over the world and from different walks of life found ways to work and live together.

I made a mental note to check it out sometime soon and even had the crazy thought that, one day, maybe I could try to get on that show—just to have a new experience under my belt if nothing else. Naturally, I had no idea just how soon that would happen.

In the meantime, we pushed north. Our lush surroundings gave way to harsher and more desolate environs composed mostly of ice and rock. We changed from summer clothes into thermals and coats since we had traveled from summer to winter in the span of a couple of days.

As one of our first stops past Norway, we anchored at Bear Island. Made famous as a prominent *Game of Thrones* shooting location, the island is populated with polar bears that cross to the island from the mainland when the water is frozen over and become somewhat stranded there when the ice thaws.

Seeing polar bears up close and in person like that struck me as one of the most unbelievable experiences of my life. Their indescribable magnificence caused my breath to catch in my throat as I took in the incredible sight. It's beyond anything you could even imagine.

From there, we hired an icebreaker to lead the way, and we made for the ice of Svalbard.

~

At this point, as we approached literally uncharted territory, I marveled at the way life was unfolding. All I had learned about the control

I had over my world seemed to be proven truer with every passing mile of this expedition.

When given a night shift, I would ordinarily go straight to bed, knowing I needed to be awake again in just a few hours for more work. However, I'd pulled a night shift the night before we were supposed to reach Svalbard, and I wanted to make sure I was on deck to see it the moment we came within sight. So, when my shift ended, I chose to stay awake.

This turned into one of the only all-nighters I've ever truly enjoyed in my life. Back when I partied every weekend away, I hated the feeling of the sun coming up after spending the whole night awake. But this time, as the sun began to rise, slowly illuminating the exquisite scenery, I caught the first view of Svalbard. We could have been on another planet, so extreme was the sharp change in the landscape. Temperatures dropped so low that water on the boat froze within seconds. It was *awesome.*

The next few days that we spent in Svalbard felt almost like visiting space for how otherworldly the setting had become, not to mention the surreal nature of the experience. The family who owned the yacht donned full submersion suits and went swimming under the ice. On the surface, we hiked glaciers, and when we came upon waterfalls, we stripped down to our underwear and danced in what felt like the purest, coldest natural water on planet Earth.

We met a couple living in a desolate, remote area surviving on nothing but the elements as they conducted research on the environment. They also had husky dogs, a breed that I've always loved, as my grandmother had a few when I was growing up in South Africa. Now, I was getting to see these beautiful canines in their most natural environment.

About a week and a half after first reaching Svalbard, we pushed far enough past the island to, indeed, reach our goal destination. We made it farther north than any luxury superyacht had ever gone.

All this time, I'd known I was participating in a once-in-a-lifetime experience with this expedition, and as we reached this point, I felt as though I'd absolutely squeezed everything out of it.

By the end of the expedition, we had covered 7,500 nautical miles and visited ten different countries. Perhaps best of all, we all hailed from different parts of the globe, which I found as epic and beautiful as all the physical beauty we'd encountered in our journey. Our many wildly different emotional worlds had merged on that yacht. We'd found ways to ensure our strengths and weaknesses complemented one another, and we'd created a fantastic voyage together.

The expedition had begun with me feeling humbled by being the low man on the totem pole, and now, this far north, I felt an even deeper sense of insignificance in the best possible way. Being here in this isolated, pure world within our world, I realized all over again just how small my life and my problems were in the grand scheme of things.

When I'd felt stuck in my job back home in JoBurg, every problem had seemed so big, and I'd been consumed by my own little universe, chasing money and stimulation and parties so much that I didn't have time to recognize how much I was missing out on elsewhere. Here, now, I still appreciated the work I had left to do on myself, but this gave me an unforgettable reminder of my place in the universe—and, along with that, the endless beauty to be experienced in this world.

At the same time, somehow, the scenery also evoked an incredible sense of less is more. The world was now all white from the ice and snow against the brown from the earth and the blue of the sky. This backdrop made me feel like I was living inside a work of art. No matter what troubles I faced or how hard life became, this showed me that life also always had plenty waiting for me to look forward to.

# CHAPTER 13

Within a few weeks of returning to Vlissingen, Netherlands (the location of *The Gene Machine's* shipyard), the artic expedition was done, and I was sent back home. My visa was expiring; therefore, I could not stay in Europe any longer. This was one of the biggest challenges finding permanent work for South Africans. While home, I received several new job offers, but I had to decline them because they all needed me to start immediately, and I hadn't gotten a new visa yet. My goal back home was to acquire a five- or ten-year visa that would allow me to return to Europe for a longer period of time and find more permanent work. Now that I had such an impressive experience to add to my CV after *The Gene Machine* expedition, I was hopeful finding new work should be much easier.

Since the visa would take at least a couple of months to be approved, I crashed with an uncle near the beach, lived off of my earnings from the expedition, visited with friends and family, and used the time to process everything I had just experienced. People don't even get to take vacations like the expedition I'd just completed, and I'd gotten paid to do it. I felt so grateful and fortunate as well as awestruck at how everything I'd worked so diligently to implement within myself had actually paid off. I'd done the hard work of improving my subconscious mind to believe that a bigger life was possible—and then I had actually lived that bigger life.

After that experience, I realized I didn't just want my next yachting job. I wanted another opportunity to continue my personal development and growth. My goal remained the same as it had been when I'd first set out for the South of France: take my life to the next level.

One day that November, while catching up on the phone with a friend from the South of France, he mentioned that he'd been approached by producers of a reality television series called *Below Deck.* That reminded me of my conversation with one of my crewmates aboard *The Gene Machine,* and I told my friend that I'd thought about possibly pursuing a spot on the show someday myself. Without hesitation, he offered to put me right in touch with one of the show's recruiters, so I figured what the hell! I was looking for work, and if there was an outside chance at landing my next job as part of a reality television show, then that would likely offer an incredible experience of a very different kind.

I didn't expect much to happen right away, but after the recruiter received my CV, he quickly scheduled an interview by video chat. As I realized that this could be a real possibility, I decided that this was the next logical step in my journey. I began to feel the same sense of confidence in my desire for this to happen as I had felt when I'd first started making plans for the South of France.

As the interview began, I naturally experienced some nerves and uncertainty, but I just reminded myself that this was another exciting opportunity. The questions seemed designed to gauge whether I would make for good entertainment value while also being a hard worker. In addition, the interview focused on how my personality would fit with the other cast members they were considering.

Things moved surprisingly swiftly from there. I reminded myself that all I really had to do was just be my best, most charming, most charismatic self.

And I loved it. I had good experience, I'd learned a lot, I had a likable personality, and I felt hungry for more. We shared some banter, told some jokes, and made each other laugh. I answered all their questions as truthfully as I could—and, mostly, I just had fun with the interview, trusting that my personality would shine through.

Then, in the first or second week of January, a producer called and told me they'd selected me to be a member of their cast for the upcoming season. Shooting would begin at the end of February.

How wild was this? Just over a year prior to this, I'd been stuck with no clear sense of direction for my life. Now, I was being offered a position on an American reality television show. Once again, I found myself facing the unknown, and still, I found security in that unknown. Accordingly, I resolved that even though I had no idea what waited for me next, I would find something that would help me continue to take my life to the next level.

That said, I didn't realize the magnitude of *Below Deck* at the time. All I knew was that it was a reality show based around working on yachts. I'd never watched it. I was just grateful to have another good job again, and I was looking forward to a new experience. It felt like the next step up in my life. Coming off a three-month expedition through Europe and the Arctic, I knew it was unrealistic to expect my next experience to top that, but I figured joining the cast of a reality television show gave me as good of a chance at that as possible.

The producers sent over a contract, which I signed immediately. The pay was slightly more than when I was working on *The Gene Machine,* so I was perfectly pleased with that. Everything happened so quickly, I barely took time to peruse the contract. In hindsight, I wish I'd read it more closely, but if I'm being honest, I would've signed it anyway—I just didn't realize exactly what I was signing up for. Nevertheless, like everything else I do in my life, by this point, I had already committed to throwing myself one thousand percent into this next process.

Since this season of the show would be shooting in Tahiti, I embarked on a mad scramble with the French Consulate to acquire my new visa for French Polynesia. The producers helped me move quickly through that process. Then, the next thing I knew, I'd booked a plane ticket to Tahiti.

Once again, everything kept falling into place.

Up until the moment I sat down on the plane, I'd been so in get-shit-done mode that I hadn't taken the time to fully process what was actually happening. After I took my seat, things got real. I was about to be on an American reality television show watched by over a million people.

*What the hell?* I thought. *Is this really my life?*

I just kept cycling through thoughts and memories of where I had been not so long ago and what I now had waiting for me next. If you apply yourself and put yourself out there, big things really can happen for you and your life.

And then . . . some anxiety began to kick in about what, exactly, *was* waiting for me next. I was also acutely aware of the fact that I wasn't exactly a seasoned yachtsman. With less than a full year's worth of experience under my belt, and having only served one real contract out at sea, I still felt like barely more than a greenie in the industry. Now, I was on a plane bound for Tahiti, where I would be putting my skills to the test for an audience of more than a million.

*Holy shit,* I thought. *Do you actually know what you're getting yourself into?*

Working a yacht felt fun and glamorous at times, to be sure, but also required consistent focus and performance during high-stress situations—even without a camera crew in your face. Could I handle that sort of scrutiny and still do my job well? Or would I choke under the pressure and somehow screw up something major? This could easily make my career for years to come—but it also suddenly seemed as though it could destroy my career for good if I messed up badly enough.

As the plane carried me over the Pacific toward Tahiti, my mind brought every insecurity and weakness I thought I had to the surface. Finally, however, I calmed myself down, same as in the interviews, telling myself once again to just be myself. Find security in the unknown—all of the unknown.

No, I absolutely did not know what I was getting myself into. But I could trust myself to handle things properly, and if mistakes occurred, I could trust myself to make them right and learn from the experience, no matter what happened.

The nerves faded. Peace returned. And with the peace came confidence and joy and excitement.

Besides, how much could go wrong, really?

# CHAPTER 14

Upon landing in Tahiti, I found a car and driver waiting for me at the airport to take me to my hotel, where I was sneaked in through a side door, everything very cloak and dagger to ensure no cast members met each other before shooting began.

The hotel was nice and comfortable with everything I could need. As it rained nonstop outside, I used my time to Google Tahiti and French Polynesia and daydreamed about what could happen next—what it would be like acclimating to a new job and new crew while also having television cameras in our faces the whole time. Having zero experience on camera, and being a shy person by nature, I had a feeling that would be . . . uncomfortable to say the least.

Finally, it was time to go. Producers took us to the boat one at a time. My guess was that they'd waited for the rain to clear out because, when they took me out of the hotel, the weather was perfect. Clear skies, lovely temperature, a slight breeze, the scent of saltwater in the air mixing wonderfully with the smell of fresh rain—a beautiful day.

Approaching the boat, I saw more producers, along with a half-dozen cameramen and their cameras on deck, giving me the sense that I wasn't just boarding a yacht but also stepping foot onto some sort of massive television set. And with that, I also felt a jolt of anxiety. The yacht was already huge, and when you added in the whole production crew on board, the situation felt somewhat overwhelming.

But as I boarded the boat and began to introduce myself to everybody, I felt a switch flip in me. Yes, I felt nervous due to my minor yacht experience—and nonexistent television experience—but this was a real job, and not just for me. All of those producers and cameramen had a job to do and a quality television show to make too. Their eyes might have all been on me, but they also relied on me following their instructions and fulfilling my role as a television cast member. One of their most important instructions had been to never break the fourth wall by looking directly at or addressing a camera at all, so I had to find a way to forget about the lenses winking at me from various directions.

Beyond the television crew, my fellow yacht crewmates probably also felt similar emotions—probably harbored the same concerns about making mistakes and had the same desire to be part of a good show. None of us wanted to look like an idiot in front of a million people. We could make the biggest mistake in the world, and they could cut it out of the show entirely. Or we could do everything perfectly except for one thing, and that one error could still be witnessed by hundreds of thousands of viewers. No amount of worrying about cameras or producers would have any effect on how we were presented to the show's audience.

We had no control over anything except how we conducted ourselves and did our jobs. With that in mind, I remembered, once again, to simply surrender and find security in the unknown.

Day one was all about settling into the yacht and getting to know the crew. Captain Lee had white hair with matching white beard, a fatherly disposition, and little patience for bullshit. He quickly gave me an impression of a good captain who clearly had ample experience in the industry, and he naturally gave and commanded respect in equal measure.

With no time to waste, the very next day, everything kicked into high gear as our first guests were coming aboard and our initial charter would begin. That meant it was time to go to work—and it was show-time. Our new uniforms on and cameras all around, we welcomed the guests with warmth and smiles, doing our best to act as though we all knew each other as a crew and trying to pretend like there weren't cameras everywhere we turned. We helped the guests settle into the yacht, ensuring they all felt happy and were having a good time. Then, Captain Lee fired up the engines, and we dropped the lines and made our way out of port.

Despite having spent less than twenty-four hours aboard the yacht, we already found ourselves at sea. Tahiti was nothing like I'd ever seen back in the Mediterranean, especially the massive reefs surrounding the main island. We tried to behave as though we weren't still getting our bearings, simply doing our jobs and accommodating the guests as though we'd done this forever, despite the fact that we were still getting to know the boat and the environment, not to mention each other as well.

Having cameras in my face the entire time made it quite challenging to have an authentic conversation and create a genuine connection with strangers, even though they were now my crewmates for the coming season. Everyone else was just as aware of the cameras as I was, so it was difficult to let my guard down enough to feel like someone was seeing the real me, and it was hard to feel out the people I was meeting too. I kept wondering if I was talking to who this person really was or if this was just who they wanted to present to the camera—and I tried to make sure that I wasn't presenting a false version of myself just because *I* knew we were on camera.

I did hit it off pretty quickly with one crew member—my bunk-mate, Ross, the lead deckhand and someone who struck me as sincere and good-hearted from the start. A native New Zealander, he'd also played a lot of rugby. Our two countries were famous for being rugby powerhouses and rivals in the sport, and we realized that our upbringings and backgrounds also shared a number of traits. We clicked from that first day aboard, quickly starting to banter back and forth, and he would go on to become one of my good friends the more we got to know each other. In him, I felt I'd found a brother and we'd have each other's backs.

Then, there was the work itself. I realized that my ever-present mentality of always working like somebody was watching was now my complete and total reality. Somebody really *was* always watching. And recording. And the things they recorded could potentially be broadcast to a million people.

Can you imagine? Just doing your job, knowing that countless people could be watching your every move, listening to your every conversation, seeing every expression that crossed your face when your boss gave you orders you may have had less-than-pleasant feelings about?

And not just your job, but your time off too—when you go out with your friends to the pub or spend time with your family or do whatever else it is that you enjoy in your free time? There were cameras in our kitchen, our lounge—even our bunk rooms had little night vision cameras tucked up and away in the corners. Producers would be watching us *sleep* in our *beds*—not to mention whatever else can and often does happen in beds.

Can you imagine cameras on you virtually every moment of every day?

Being watched *all the time* felt like so much more of a huge thing than I could have possibly anticipated. As our season began, I tried to tell myself to just ignore the cameras, do my job, and be myself, but life became a constant battle between, *Okay, I'm just going to focus on getting the job done,* and, *Holy shit, there are cameras all around us.*

As I would see later, some crew members simply couldn't handle the constant scrutiny. And truthfully, acclimating took me quite some time. I found myself constantly second- and triple- and quadruple-guessing myself. Performing my tasks and simply moving about the yacht while feeling natural and confident felt almost impossible. Every instinct I had and every bit of conditioning I'd developed over the course of my life suddenly felt thrown into question. With each line I tied, with each conversation I had, I found my mind wondering: *Is this the right way to do this? Is this the right thing to say right now? Is my face being the right . . . face?*

But same as when I'd first gone aboard *The Gene Machine,* I entered this situation by recognizing my role and respecting my place in the pecking order. As a junior deckhand, I was once again essentially at the bottom of the totem pole with less yachting experience than anyone else on board except for a woman named Rhylee, my fellow junior deckhand. And as a reality television cast member, all of this was brand new to me.

I reminded myself to approach this season the same way I'd approached last year's Arctic expedition—by keeping my head down, handling my responsibilities, doing whatever my superiors asked of me without question or complaint, and doing all I could to make everyone else's lives aboard the yacht better.

After leaving port and making our way out to sea, we traveled through a narrow channel with reefs beneath us and large, sweeping waves rising and falling on both sides of the yacht. Upon emerging on the other side of the channel, we arrived in a small cove, a haven of calm water. We would spend our first day and first night here. Captain Lee dropped anchor, and then all the toys came out.

Quickly, our number one concern became keeping the guests safe due to the endless supply of reefs throughout the water. While we encouraged them to have fun on the toys—the jet skis were a particularly in-demand item—we had to strike a proper balance by ensuring that they operated them the right way without putting themselves in danger.

Some of the guests had never driven a jet ski before, and all of them swiftly reached various levels of intoxication. Sure enough, that first day, one of the guests was going nuts on a jet ski and went zooming into a reef. In the collision, he was sent flying. We raced to tend to him, trying to conceal our panic from both the guests and the cameras, and were relieved to discover that he was, somehow, entirely unharmed. Despite our gratitude at confirming his health, I found the incident a fitting encapsulation of just how quickly this entire situation had become overwhelming.

Keep in mind, the guests were *also* hyperaware of the cameras, which could make them nervous. They could compensate for that by acting over-confident—or simply showing off. While that certainly makes for good entertainment, it can also put people in dangerous situations.

Particularly after this harrowing experience, I realized there was so much more to this job than I could have first imagined. On one hand, I had to be hyper-focused—to the point of feeling stressed—to ensure everyone's safety. At the same time, I had to refrain from putting that stress on any of the guests while ensuring they all had a good time and generally maintaining good vibes for everyone involved. Even a minor moment of tension or frustration that I expressed *away* from the guests *might* be caught on camera, so that was always something to keep in mind too.

By the end of the first charter, as we returned to port, saw our guests off, and completed our duties on the yacht, I felt every emotion you can imagine: exhaustion, relief, excitement, and my ever-present disbelief at the highlight reel that my life had become. More than anything, I wanted to blow off some steam.

The rest of the crew felt the same. Our first night after that charter, we left the yacht for a night on the town. We went to dinner at a restaurant, then indulged in drinks and dancing at a club, same as any other crew working any other yacht on a night off—except for the entourage of cameramen and producers following in our wake.

The thought crossed my mind that maybe this was why reality television shows always featured so much drama. Something about cameras following us everywhere and knowing we were being watched every second had a magnifying effect on every emotion that we felt.

By the time we were in the club a few drinks deep, I felt myself begin to settle into having a good time. I was in a new place, around new people, on the island of Tahiti in French Polynesia—life was pretty freaking great. I remembered that, despite the cameras, I could let go of the pressure and the anxiety I'd been carrying. Now that I was able to let loose a bit, I reminded myself that I was a fun guy and a good worker, and I loved what I was doing. I could just let all of that emerge and stop worrying how it might all play out on television.

The alcohol flowed, we all relaxed more and overthought less, and soon enough, I started feeling like my old self, getting caught up in the night and all the fun it had to offer. The cameras actually started to make things fun, as a matter of fact, because everywhere we went, the locals would stop and turn and stare, trying to figure out who we were and what the cameras were all about. Cool men and women alike wanted to join the party. We started feeling sort of like VIPs.

I was having such a good time drinking and meeting new people, dancing and generally partying my face off. Inevitably, when the rest of the crew decided to return to the boat, I wasn't ready to go. The night was far too young to end. In our collective drunken state, this led to a hilarious argument over whether we should call it a night. Of course, I ended up sticking with my crew in the end.

The next morning, some of them told me that they hadn't appreciated the way I'd handled things and that I had sort of pissed them off. I felt bad about that and apologized sincerely. Ultimately, it turned out to be a funny joke between us all—and it certainly wasn't the last time we'd all have ourselves a big, drunken night on the town.

*Below Deck* kept every charter to around three days each, and after two or three charters, I started forgetting about the cameras as I kept my focus on adapting to my job and doing it well. Ross and I continued getting along and bantering easily, and having a good friend like that working with me during this crazy experience helped to take the edge off on more challenging days.

Another aspect to working on a yacht is that, sometimes, the experience can become rather lonely. While shooting *Below Deck,* I found that to be especially true. The situation always contained some sort of conflict or drama, and that quickly created a draining environment that could feel isolating.

If you've watched the show, then you likely know what I'm talking about. If you haven't watched the show, I'll provide an overview without sharing too much detail. Our bosun, Chandler, new to reality television, began having a hard time. He clashed with some of the other crew members as he navigated the overall pressure that comes with running a yacht. Clearly, he was genuinely trying his best at the job, and the new environment gave him a great deal to get used to. Sometimes, that could become difficult and frustrating. Our chief stew[9], Kate, was a yachting and reality television veteran at this point, and she took issue with Chandler at times due to his leadership style.

In addition, my fellow junior deckhand Rhylee's personality began to emerge more and more as time went on. To be more specific, she had a very strong personality that led her to also start sparring with Chandler. Her background before *Below Deck* was in working fishing boats, not charter yachts, and while I know nothing about working on fishing boats, her behavior on our yacht began to create a great deal of stress for everyone on deck and left me feeling deeply confused. When Chandler would give orders for various work tasks, Rhylee often rolled her eyes, sighed or groaned, presented poor body language, and generally gave the impression that, at any moment, she might explode. Sometimes, she would, becoming confrontational to the point of insubordinate anytime she felt like she was being disrespected.

---

9 The chief stew is in charge of the crew that works the interior of a yacht, handling duties such as laundry, cooking, cleaning, and the like.

Over the course of a couple more charters, the tension between Rhylee and Chandler continued to build. At a certain point, guests began picking up on it, and the rest of us found ourselves sort of tiptoeing around, trying not to add any more fuel to this steadily growing wildfire. And then, eventually—in hindsight, inevitably—an eruption finally happened. Rhylee began screaming and shouting at Chandler over something, and he responded by screaming and shouting back.

Then, this cycle repeated itself.

This was so perplexing to me because, in my experience, having to accept orders or tones of voice that were unpleasant at times simply came with the territory of being a junior deckhand. You should expect to be given respect, but you should also know your place in the pecking order. I found myself imagining what it would have been like to have someone like Rhylee aboard *The Gene Machine* during our expedition and felt that she likely would have been removed from the boat rather quickly. I had a hard time imagining how else things would go in the real world.

This began to make me feel more baffled than ever—to the point where I began doubting my own values and all that I had learned in my previous yachting experience. As far as I knew, this sort of thing simply never happened on yachts, or if it did, it would only happen one time and then never again.

Typically, one of two things occurs after even one explosion like the many Rhylee and Chandler kept having. One, the two people have a calm conversation in which they sort out their issues and find a new understanding of each other, leading to a respectful resolution that reestablishes a healthy work environment. Two, as a result of uncompromising animosity and conflict between the two people, one simply gets fired from the boat—usually the subordinate failing to give their superior the proper deference and respect.

But now, I was starting to question what I knew. Was this sort of behavior actually normal and I was just struggling to accept it? I had a hard time believing that could be possible because the situation felt increasingly unproductive and uncomfortable, but I couldn't help but consider alternatives. Should I be more tolerant and understanding of Rhylee's attitude? Was my experience on *The Gene Machine* actually just a stroke of luck in how that crew and expedition matched my personal values? Was the sort of thing happening here and now what usually happened on other yachts? Was this really acceptable?

Maybe, I figured, this was just part of the magic of *Below Deck*—the way they brought all these different individuals together and let them bounce off of one another. When you put a bunch of people with strong personalities in a high-pressure environment like this, that drama becomes largely inescapable. While such behavior is the perfect example of what you don't want to have on a boat, I suppose that's the special sauce for reality television.

As the season carried on, the cameramen certainly recorded plenty the producers could work with. Beyond his ongoing conflict with Rhylee, the deck crew as a whole lacked the correct guidance and leadership from Chandler. While I sympathized with the challenges he had on his plate, we still had a boat to run, and the "show" needed to go on. Ultimately, about halfway through the season, Captain Lee decided that the best thing for everyone would be to let Chandler go. Having been overwhelmed, even Chandler agreed with the decision, expressed relief when it was made, and left in peace.

Ross was appointed new bosun, I took over Ross's role as lead deckhand, and Captain Lee hired a new junior deckhand named Tyler. He turned out to be a cool, fun guy with sailing experience who regularly worked as a firefighter. With his chill vibe and fun attitude, he gave our crew a breath of fresh air after all the conflict and drama.

Right around this time, things began to change for the better. Rhylee abruptly became more relaxed, and her attitude was much more positive and cooperative. In fact, she became downright bubbly, bouncing around the deck, getting work done, and literally no longer arguing at all.

What had shifted? Well, best as we could all tell, this change began taking place around the same time that Rhylee began hooking up with

Tyler. We joked with her about this. *Damn, Rhylee, all you needed was to be getting some?* I was sincerely glad for her, though, because she seemed so much happier.

Usually, when people are so angry, there is something deeply rooted that needs attention, and I have compassion for people in these situations. After all, I have a lot of the same thing that I am dealing with.

Better still, her improved demeanor had a remarkable effect on crew morale all around. Everyone began to get along super well, and we became a more cohesive and productive crew than ever. We had more fun together, and the entire vibe aboard the yacht shifted into something that felt like what this whole experience should have always been about. Yes, we had to work hard, and yes, that hard work was often unpleasant, but ultimately, even the most unpleasant aspects of the job became the most rewarding. After all, when we were finished with the work, we were aboard a luxury superyacht off the coast of freakin' Tahiti. What was there to complain about?

Even if I didn't always like the orders Ross gave me or agree with everything he said, I felt a lot of respect for him in the bosun position due to his experience. Ross had been in the yachting industry for about five years by that point, and while he had become a close friend, in some ways, he also felt like a mentor with much to teach me. He always seemed humble and ready to answer any questions as well as help me learn anything I might not know. We continued with our banter but also cultivated a mutual respect for each other. In a way, Ross took me under his wing, but he never treated me as though he was somehow better than me in any way. Given all the challenges inherent to our situation, having him there as a friend and a brother whom I felt understood what was going on provided a nice bit of comfort.

But then, the same conflicts started to arise between Rhylee and Ross, and her behavior toward him gradually mirrored her behavior toward Chandler. They began to experience the same cycle that Chandler had also experienced with Rhylee.

I started to feel so bewildered all over again. Talking with Ross about it along the way, I finally voiced my confusion about the whole situation. When I wondered if I should just let this go because it was normal, he affirmed to me that things with Rhylee were indeed unusual and not the way conflict was typically handled aboard a yacht.

"She's just too much," he said at one point. "She did this with Chandler, and now she's doing this with me. We need somebody else in here that's going to be a team player and put being productive for the team as their first priority."

In many ways, Rhylee was valuable. She had a number of strengths, chief among them her strong work ethic. She knew how to work hard. On the other hand, she also kept taking everything personally, almost as though she were looking for reasons to be angry and upset, and she was very difficult to get along with. She just seemed to enjoy fighting. As time went on, her ego seemed to grow larger and larger, and we all found ourselves trying to tiptoe around it. This became exhausting. We already got little sleep many nights, we were in a high-pressure situation, and every bit of our energy was being spent on navigating that while keeping our shit together. The work itself wore us out—and then we had a personality like this to contend with as well.

So, those were the things on Ross's mind that he pointed out to me, and that helped clarify expectations a bit. After three or four weeks of this, he was actually feeling so stressed by the situation that he was considering asking Captain Lee to have Rhylee removed from the boat as well. The tension had escalated so much between them that Ross felt anxiety every time he had to ask Rhylee to do anything, even simple, basic orders.

The renewed tension and conflict started to take its toll on everyone. Then, as if that weren't enough, something even more significant happened—and it happened to me.

It started out just like any other guest arrival day. The guests arrived at the shipyard around midday, and we welcomed them aboard the yacht. As they came on board, they met Captain Lee and the crew, and just like that, it was time to get the party started.

After we brought the guests' luggage on board and took them to their respective cabins, our next mission was to get the yacht off the dock. There are three key steps for this to happen.

First, the captain gives orders on which lines he wants dropped, and the crew has to drop those as quickly as possible. Once all lines are on deck, the captain is informed so he knows that nothing's holding him to the dock anymore, and it's all in his control.

Stage two is helping him navigate out of port. For that to happen, somebody on the bow and somebody on the aft must call out distances to help the captain envision where he needs to maneuver the boat to safely exit the port. This involves calling out things that the captain can't see from his position and getting him clear of any obstructions so he can cruise out of the channel.

The third part is when the crew releases the tender off the hip and gets it on tow safely behind the boat. This is a high-pressure situation because, if the setup of that line is incorrect, it can mess up the entire maneuver and put everyone in a compromising position, especially with being in the channel. If the captain can't keep continuous control and direction of the boat in the direction that it needs to go, and the crew has to stop and address hooked lines, it can quickly become a dangerous situation.

Things were going well enough as we initiated the first step. Riley and Ross were on the aft while Tyler and I took up our positions on the bow. At this point, the engines were started, and we were just waiting for the captain to give us word on which lines he wanted detached first.

To help you visualize this, I'm going to give you a quick crash course in how this all works. When we unravel the lines from the cleats in the boat, it creates slack in the line. People on the dock, like the dock masters, then unloop the line from the cleat that's connected to the dock. After that, we pull as hard and quick as possible on those lines to get them back onto the boat.

Now, there are a lot more lines than there are deckhands. So, we've got to be very systematic with which lines we release first. Obviously, when we release the lines, the boat starts moving and drifting off the dock. So, the way the wind is blowing determines which lines are released first. For example, if a wind is hitting the back of the boat, pushing the boat forward, then we are going to leave the line that's holding the boat, preventing it from moving forward, for last. Otherwise, the wind will push us into a potentially hazardous position before we get all the lines off, which will make controlling the boat off the dock a lot harder for the captain.

By this point, we were quite proficient at all this, and after receiving direction from the captain, we promptly released all the lines that we needed and got them on deck. I remained on the bow for the next stage, calling out distances to the captain, and we made our way toward the end of the channel.

Feeling grateful to have accomplished that swiftly and smoothly, I decided to go to the aft deck to see if I could help Ross and Riley for that tricky third phase. This is where things went sideways.

Now, before we started this whole procedure, before we even got the guests on the boat, we had a tow line pre-set up onto the two very aft cleats on the swim platform at the back of the boat. Once we'd secured it around the cleats, we coiled the line in such a manner that it wasn't going to tangle when the boat was released behind so that it could self-uncoil.

This was incredibly important for us to safely and smoothly exit the channel. Think about it this way: If we just ran a line from the back of the boat, coiled it, and then put it to the front of the tender, there would be slack, and that that line would hang in the water. That's bad because there are propellers at the back of the boat, and there's a chance of the line being sucked under and getting wrapped in the propellers. So, to eliminate that last bit of slack between the coil on the swim platform and the front of the tender, it's crucial to pull the line through one of the cleats up on the aft deck, then tie it off on a cleat so that the tender's nice and tight against the yacht, and there's no slack in the water.

As I was coming down the deck toward Riley and Ross, looking to help them with this delicate maneuver, the pair released the front line off the midship cleat and tossed it into the tender. That allowed the tender to start drifting back. From there, the captain thrusted to move the boat in the opposite direction to the tender, and the wash of the propellers kicked it away from the yacht. As the captain hit the boat into forward gear, ensuring the tender was away from the yacht and drifting back, the coil that was set up on the swim platform started feeding out.

While all this played out, I noticed the line was hooked around one of the fenders in between the tender and the yacht. So, I went down onto the swim platform, diligently attempting to rectify the problem.

That was my first mistake. One should never be on the swim platform when this line is being paid out. However, someone had to get the line hooked off the fender; otherwise, it would have just ripped the fender off the boat. So, I decided to just unhook the line, noting there was still enough slack in it for it not to be super dangerous. As I did that, the tender was still paying out, and I just followed the line, making sure it wasn't hooked on anything else.

Meanwhile, Riley was next to me, and I was reminding her, "Watch the line, watch the line. Stay back, stay back." Even as I was saying that to her, I wasn't doing it myself. Do as I say it, not as I do, right?

At this stage, a good part of that line had already fed out into the water, and the tender was already drifting back at quite a decent speed. Keep in mind, the further along in this maneuver you get, the faster things start happening because the yacht's building up momentum, and the tender's building up momentum moving backwards as well. So, what had once been a relatively harmless action was rapidly becoming decidedly unsafe . . .

As I was holding the line in my hand, I felt a mighty tug on my ankle. That's when I looked down and realized my grave error.

Looking at Rhylee in shock, I knew instantly what was to come. "I'm going in," I said.

"No," she said, lunging for me. "No, no, no."

Rhylee reached out, trying to save me, but there was nothing she could do. In an instant, as the tender continued to release from the yacht, that line pulled away with uncontrollable force. In the space of a heartbeat, I recognized that I was going in, so I tried to put myself in the best situation possible to release myself once I hit the water.

I plunged in feet first. My eyes stung as I fought to sneak the occasional gasp of air while grappling with the line. For several futile moments, I struggled underwater to release my ankle from the impossibly tight loop, but it was no use.

At the time, all I could think was, *I'm gonna lose my foot.* You know, you hear of people losing fingers and hands and stuff on yachts, but you never think it's going to happen to you. Yet there I was, wildly thinking, *I am about to become a statistic. My foot is about to be ripped off at the ankle.*

Later, I would reflect on the gruesome reality of what could have happened. See, nobody would be able to get to me in time to save me from the physical trauma of losing my foot. So, I would've just bled out in the water. Yep—I was facing death, but in that moment, I wasn't thinking about that brutal consequence. I just knew my foot was going to be rendered from my body, and there was nothing I could do about it.

I screamed, gutturally releasing all the fear and pain and pitching headfirst into full acceptance of whatever horror awaited me next.

I'd never been in a situation like this where I had to accept something so horrific and life-changing happening to me. The scream ripping from my throat was more desperate and primal than any sound that had ever erupted from my body. It felt like I was screaming *for* my life.

But then . . . Just as my scream died . . . As if by a miracle . . .

I felt relief. Total and utter relief. And I don't mean just in the metaphysical, spiritual sense. I mean the line had gone slack. My foot now drifted safely down into the sea with me.

*I was free.*

# CHAPTER 15

*Oh my god. What just happened?*

Looking back at the yacht, I saw people standing on the deck and realized that somebody had somehow released the line from the cleat on the yacht. Ross was calling out to me, asking if I was okay. I raised my hand, giving a sign that I was.

I felt dazed by the whole situation, but that moment burned itself into my mind forever. After finding myself drowning and moments from dismemberment, after being pushed to the point of accepting my physical form was about to be torn asunder, in the very instant that I actually found the capacity to surrender to that reality—I was spared.

There was little time to bask in such profundities, however. For all my spiritualizing, I remained very human, and I still had a job to do, not to mention a mess of my own making to clean up.

"Get the tender!" Ross yelled from the yacht. "Get the tender!"

Turning around, I saw the tender rapidly drifting away from the yacht and back toward the shore. That encapsulated my entire life: No matter what major incident might have just happened to me, life always came calling, saying to me, *Get up, Ashton. Time for the next thing.* There was no time to sit and cry and figure out what was going on. I had to move forward.

Ignoring the fiery, pulsating pain in my leg, I unwound the tender line and used it to pull myself rapidly toward the tender. After hauling myself aboard and piling the tender line into the boat with me, I frantically tried to get the boat to start. With my adrenaline pumping, my body was literally shaking, and I struggled to get the engine to turn over, even as I drifted further from the yacht and closer to the rocks ashore. I'd gone from one panicked situation right into another. Between the trauma of what I'd just experienced and the adrenaline coursing through my veins, my brain was simply all over the place.

Radioing Ross, I told him I had no idea what to do. He talked me through some options, such as checking the kill switch and the ignition and a few other things. After what felt like an eternity, the engine finally started.

Captain Lee radioed in, telling me he was glad that I was okay and to just follow the yacht in the tender until we reached anchorage.

While piloting the tender, as my adrenaline gradually faded and my ankle started throbbing violently, I began to experience an intense cycle of emotions. I'd feel calm and grateful to have survived, then swing into extreme anxiety over what had just happened, overthinking everything about it and questioning everything about myself. That would transform into anger directed at myself, as I felt so stupid for having put myself in that situation at all. I also worried about the consequences I'd face for my carelessness when I returned to the yacht, all but certain I'd lose my job because I'd completely ruined this entire experience, even for other members of the crew and our guests. Then, boom, I'd be calm again, and the cycle would repeat.

Our trip to anchorage took around forty minutes, and the solo tender ride gave me a nice way to work through those emotions and start to process what had just happened. Had I been taken straight back aboard the yacht, I would have been overwhelmed by everyone checking on me and fussing over me. This way, I had space to begin to feel what I had to feel and move past judging myself for what had happened.

Checking my ankle, I saw imprints from where the line had gripped me, carved deep and painful, red and blue and purple, into my skin, little dermatological canyons winding their way around my leg. I wondered just how badly broken things were under the surface.

After reaching anchorage, when I returned aboard, Ross met me first, embracing me with a tight hug and tears in his eyes. That moment felt like returning home. I felt so grateful for him, for our friendship, and for the comfort that brought me now. Then, like any good brother, he told me to never let anything that stupid happen to me again. "You scared the shit out of me," he said.

What happened next has become something of a blur in my memory. At some point, I learned the reason the line had gone slack: A hero had saved me. One of the cameramen on the aft deck had acted quickly, throwing down his camera and going for the line, freeing it from the cleat just in time and releasing it into the sea.

But the show had to go on, of course—we still had guests on board. The crew returned to their duties as I went to my cabin to nurse my ankle. Captain Lee came down to check on me, seeming a bit shaken and expressing just how relieved he was that I was okay. He knew that these things happened sometimes, and any concerns I'd had about him being upset with me were squashed by how kind and caring he was toward me.

A doctor was brought aboard to examine my foot, and amazingly, she determined that while there was deep bruising, some trauma to my Achilles heel, and ample swelling, nothing was actually broken. We wrapped the ankle and iced it. Other than that, all I could do for the time being was rest and recover.

This drove me bonkers, of course, because I felt terrible just lying in my bunk while the rest of the crew had to run a charter a full man down. I kept my radio on, trying to feel like part of the action even in that small way by listening to what everyone was doing.

Ross checked on me whenever he had a break and gave me updates on how things were going. Kate kindly brought me meals. Rhylee and Tyler kept popping in, too, asking if I needed anything else. Producers checked on me regularly as well. In some ways, the attention felt a bit embarrassing, but in other ways, this deepened that sense of belonging that I loved about being part of a crew. Everyone assured me that I shouldn't worry—they were just happy that I was alive and okay.

With a great deal of time to myself in my cabin as I recuperated, I continued to process my emotions about the accident and did a lot of reflection. What had happened had been a truly life-or-death situation. Working in the industry, you'll hear stories about big incidents happening on a boat, but they always feel far removed from your life, like they're not actually possible for you or anyone you know. Now, I was one of those stories. I felt lucky to be alive but also regretful for putting my crew in such a compromising position. They needed me, and I wasn't there for them, and at times, I felt deeply frustrated with myself for allowing this to happen.

Other times, however, I just felt deep gratitude for everyone on board and their commitment to being there for me. Every time somebody checked on me or brought me food or water or something, they disrupted my train of heavy thoughts and made me feel cared for. Their mere presence felt like its own dose of medicine.

On the final day of the charter, after the guests departed, we all gathered in the lounge for what we called our tip meeting. Same as every charter, we discussed how things had gone, and then Captain Lee told us how much of a cash tip the guests had left us. He then distributed the cash to each member of the crew in equal portions.

When he handed me my cash, I handed it back to him, saying that I didn't think I'd contributed enough to this trip and didn't feel right taking part of the tip, so my portion should be split up among everyone else. I felt like they deserved it because not only had they taken care of me and looked out for me, but they'd also had to pick up the extra hours I wasn't able to work and take on the extra labor I wasn't able to perform. Giving them my tip was simply the right thing to do.

Captain Lee rebuffed me immediately. "That's not how this works," he said. "You're part of the crew."

As much as that meant to me, I also determined that with a few more charters to go in this season, not another charter would pass without my contribution in one form or another, even if that meant simply washing dishes in the galley.

There was little I could do for the next couple of days, but back at port, I began attending physiotherapy. The primary task there was to do something about the swelling. An enormous amount of blood had pooled in the damaged area, putting me at risk of developing major scar tissue that could restrict my mobility. So much blood had gathered there that the area had the consistency of Play-Doh. You could press your thumb into my skin, and it would leave an indent.

My physiotherapist needed to get that blood moving so that, eventually, it would shift back out of the area rather than getting stuck there. Making that happen required deep massages on my ankle multiple times that week. Those massages were, in a word, excruciating. Imagine this part of your body has just suffered major trauma, and the way to heal said trauma isn't to leave it alone but rather to dig into it to make sure that the aftereffects don't cripple you permanently. Like I said . . . excruciating.

In the meantime, I forced myself back to work, probably sooner than my foot was ready, limping my way around the yacht. If massaging the damage kept the blood flowing and thus helped the damage heal properly, then surely a bit more light movement on my feet would do the same. I just couldn't keep lying around doing nothing.

Soon enough, I was able to return to my full duties as long as I could tolerate a bit of pain and discomfort. As the season went on, I steadily grew stronger. To aid in that recovery, I continued with my physiotherapy sessions two to three times per week, and every session included one of those lovely massages. It was necessary for me to undergo that painful process so that my injured ankle could properly heal. In many ways I couldn't possibly see at the time, this would serve as a metaphor for my life.

# CHAPTER 16

As the season concluded, I found myself feeling reflective again. Holy shit—what a season it had been, and what a path my life was taking. Everything had played out in such extreme fashion. I'd gone from making these enormous changes a year and a half ago, leaving my corporate job and setting out on this quest to become a yachtie with no clue how that would even play out. That had landed me that epic first contract on *The Gene Machine,* perhaps the most incredible first yacht experience I could have asked for.

And then, as my follow-up to that, the universe had brought me *Below Deck.* That experience had been full of drama—dramatic location, crew drama, and a near fatal incident involving . . . me! I'd built wonderful relationships with people on the crew, especially Ross, with whom I remained in contact after we parted ways, and we even made plans to visit. Along the way, I'd almost freaking lost my life.

*Like holy shit, Ashton. You know how to do things proper.*

Extreme was the word, alright.

Reflecting on all that had happened in the past two years, I felt a huge sense of gratitude and awe. You really can build a dream life for yourself if you just commit to it, believe in yourself, and trust the unexpected detours that might arise along the way. I mean, I had nearly died, and yet that had given me one of the most profound experiences of my life.

As I returned to JoBurg after *Below Deck,* I wondered how things could possibly get better than they had been—or, at least, more extreme.

~

At season's end, I returned to South Africa to manage my visa and process all I'd just experienced. Wanting some space from people and time to myself, I rented an Airbnb and spent a lot of my time alone so that I could decompress.

One day, while talking with my cousin, she asked, "Ash, have you really actually processed what happened?"

I was having a harder time dealing with my near-death experience than I'd thought. Flashbacks would hit me, and I would shake and shudder and remember, *That was a real dark moment.* I'd really thought I was about to watch my foot come off my leg. I'd thought I might bleed out and drown as a result. The fear and pain and despair of that moment would wash back over me again and again.

Having endured traumatic experiences of her own, my cousin shared some valuable insight about how she found it still affecting her from time to time, even years later. "You just have to let yourself feel it," she said.

When terrible things happen to us, when we're subjected to tremendous amounts of stress, our minds and bodies remember those moments, even if we're not constantly consciously thinking about them. They will affect us in surprising ways when we least expect it, especially if we're not properly addressing them. Little did I know at this point in my life that there were things I had experienced even before my accident that were doing exactly that—things I did not remember at the time and that I would not learn about until much later.

In the meantime, as I relaxed back home, having my cousin encourage me to pause and reflect on things was valuable guidance, and in a way, it gave me permission to actually just feel what I needed to feel. Other than my brief hiatus from work when I'd spent time journaling in the botanical gardens, I'd always moved quickly from one thing to the next, taking on one challenge after another. In many ways, I was almost living in pure survival mode. I'd never really allowed myself to just sit and simmer and consider the emotions I was experiencing and how they were affecting me.

Now, my cousin was encouraging me to be still and allow myself the time and space to feel all of the emotions that came with what had happened instead of immediately losing myself in the next experience. It was a refreshing change of pace—and one that I absolutely needed at this stage.

A few weeks after filming, *Below Deck* needed me to go shoot "pick-up" interviews with the show's producers. These are the scenes that you see in reality shows when someone is sitting in a chair discussing what is happening as it happens or reflecting on something that has happened. They film as much of this content as they can during the season itself, but there isn't always time to get everything that they need, so they do these pick-ups after the season.

And to do these, they were going to fly me to Los Angeles.

To America.

Growing up in South Africa, visiting America was everyone's pipe dream. In movies and such, the country almost didn't seem like a real place. You're told it exists, you're shown parts of it, but you never really expect to experience it for yourself.

And now, here I was, twenty-seven years old, booking a plane ticket and a hotel for my first visit to the U.S. That plane ticket and hotel was being paid for by the producers of an American television show that I'd just appeared on. And I was being flown to Los Angeles, which, to me, seemed like the land of movie stars and musicians and artists and celebrities—not to mention one of America's most iconic cities.

Suddenly, this whole *Below Deck* situation felt much, much bigger.

As I boarded the plane in JoBurg and then flew to L.A., I realized that, to this point, I still hadn't quite fully processed what it meant to be on this show. In my mind and heart, I still felt like some dude just trying to live a life that felt good for me, gave me new experiences, and helped me continue to grow and explore. Now, people were fussing over me, booking planes and cars and hotels for me. Suddenly, I was "an asset." That almost didn't feel real.

*Just stay in the moment,* I told myself. *Enjoy every second. You're getting flown to America right now to get interviewed for the television show that you're on. These are good things.*

After landing at the airport, once again, a driver awaited me with car service to take me to a hotel in Los Angeles. Once I had checked into my room, I went for a walk. Needing a haircut, I entered the first barbershop I saw, where I paid seventy dollars, having no idea whether that was expensive or not.

I would be in Los Angeles for about three days, and producers kept me on a tight schedule. While in town, in addition to filming my pick-ups, I also met with public relations firms, attending interviews with magazine journalists and radio show hosts and making various other media appearances.

Ross had flown in too since producers knew that we were friends, so we were able to spend some more time together. The work felt tiring as we talked through one scenario from the season after another for hours at a time on camera, leaving us a bit worn out for the small bit of free time we did have. Nevertheless, what a cool, surreal experience.

Over the course of the next few months, the show would fly us out there a few more times, and while we never really had the time or energy to party, we started to get better at planning ahead, had some nice evenings out at various restaurants and bars, and always made the most of our time there.

With several months to wait before *Below Deck* aired, now that I'd finished my filming and interviews for the season, I needed a job. During the season, one of the charter guests had mentioned to me that he was buying a boat and would need a crew. He'd generously said to contact him if I wanted to work for him when I finished with *Below Deck.* Thinking that landing my next gig directly off of filming the show would be ideal, I gave him a call. He said I had a job working for him if I wanted it, but I should know that the boat was in Croatia, it was much smaller than the yacht I'd been working on, and it needed a bit of work before it would be charter ready.

I'd never been to Croatia, meaning this would be a new experience. Since that was basically my chief requirement for work at this point, I said, "Let's do it." He booked my tickets, I made the necessary visa arrangements, and off I went to Croatia. After flying into the city of Split, I was greeted at the airport by the new boat's captain, a tall, skinny native Croatian who spoke broken English and seemed delighted at my arrival. Also, relieved. He and one of the boat's stewardesses took me to lunch, and then we made for the boat itself. It was docked at the Trogir Marina.

This seemed like the next wild step along my ever-unpredictable yachting journey. I'd never done "a bit of work" fixing up a boat, but I figured, how bad could it be?

As we parked the car and made for the dock, I reveled in the sharp juxtaposition between what I'd just experienced on *Below Deck*—a glamorous walk to a breathtaking yacht with a dozen crew members from a dozen different cultures—to this experience—simply me, the captain, the stewardess, and a chef. Just the four of us, three of whom barely spoke English. I loved it.

The boat would be smaller than I'd worked before, I was told, around ninety feet. I figured a smaller boat should also require less work overall. But then I saw the boat itself. It needed more than "just a bit of work"—this looked like an ancient vessel that was undergoing major renovations and was ages from being finished. Sections of the deck were missing. Various parts and pieces of equipment were scattered everywhere. The paint was dull. This yacht looked at least a year away from being ready for charter.

*What have I gotten myself into now?* I thought.

Things went from bad to worse. As we entered the inside of the boat and examined the wheelhouse, the place looked like a disaster. Charts were scattered everywhere with no clear sense of organization whatsoever. The dashboard was not only missing buttons on some of its console sections but also entire chunks of the console itself.

"Yes," the captain said. "Much work to do."

From there, we journeyed to the front of the boat to see the crew quarters, accessible by descent through a small porthole onto a tiny two-by-two-foot landing. At about ninety feet, half the size of any yacht I'd worked on thus far, the dimensions of this boat's interior left me feeling claustrophobic. To the left, we had a shower the size of an airplane toilet, and to the right, a toilet even smaller than that. Then, through a small door, I found about one foot of standing room in a space that felt like a little closet. Two sides of the wall contained cupboards. The third contained two tiny bunks. This was our cabin.

Returning to the deck, I couldn't imagine how I could possibly do what needed to be done here. I wasn't equipped for it in the slightest. All my work experience had taken place on yachts in pristine shape in luxurious, top-shelf conditions, from the yacht itself to the food served aboard to the people working on the boat. My job had been to maintain that standard of excellence. I had zero experience with restoring a yacht or with any sort of construction work for that matter. Now, I was tasked with completing an entire yacht rebuild. That would require skills I'd never used before, such as carpentry, painting, polishing, and God only knew what else.

"Listen," I said to the captain. "I don't know if I can do this."

He nodded and said that he understood, but he asked me to try the situation for just a day or two. "Let's see how that goes and then make a decision from there."

I could see the pressure he felt too. The boat needed so much work, he had very little help as it was, and his first charter was scheduled for about a month from now. Eyeing the engine parts strewn about the deck, I had no idea how we could possibly make that happen. But something about walking away felt like giving up and letting people down.

I also felt concerned that maybe I was becoming spoiled. Although, yes, I had taken a number of risks and faced a number of struggles, things had largely worked out for me thus far. I'd gotten a lot of help at the right times, and the jobs I'd landed had all been so glamorous that I felt as though I was at risk of becoming some sort of yachting snob. I'd just had two amazing jobs, the second of which had given me the VIP treatment. Now, I wanted to make sure I wasn't becoming entitled or arrogant.

Besides, in being honest with myself, I recognized the appeal in restoring this humble boat that needed so much care and attention. My bigger concern was my ability to give the boat what it needed. I knew that I would enjoy the modest nature of the small cabin, the simplicity of the work, and the solitude of being away from the heightened and engulfing experiences that I'd been having lately. Plus, I would appreciate the manual labor and the way it required me to use my hands and my physical strength.

This would be a good experience. Difficult, perhaps, but good. Everything about this job would give me new lessons and help me grow both as a yachtsman and a human being. In addition, this would give me more time and space to continue processing my near-death experience in Tahiti. It would keep me humble in my anticipation for the premier of my season of *Below Deck.* And, ultimately, it would simply give me my next challenge.

Maybe this *did* seem like an awful fit for me and my skillset, but I also wanted to believe in myself and my ability to work through that to get the job done. I'd never backed down from a challenge before and had no interest in doing so now.

I decided to stay. I would see things through.

# CHAPTER 17

Soon, I was exhausted.

Most things in life require more of you than you expect going into them, and even though I'd decided to stay in this situation expecting obstacles to overcome, somehow, the situation became even more challenging than I had expected.

That began with the captain. With a hardened, militaristic personality, an arrogant demeanor, and a habit of resorting to yelling and cursing people out, he set the tone for what often felt like a toxic environment. The contractors we'd hired to help us with some of the boat's reconstruction were frequent targets of the captain's wrath.

Other times, he shouted at me too. Soon enough, I decided to start shouting back at him. Forever grimy and dirty on this boat, physically drained by the end of every day, I found my patience for being barked at quickly expiring, so I gave it right back to him.

Interestingly, this had the unexpected effect of acting like a pressure release valve. That created a lovely pattern of working all morning while shouting at each other; sitting down for a nice, quiet lunch; and laughing about all the shit we had to do and all the shouting we were doing at each other about it. Then, we would go back to work and shout all afternoon before sharing another meal full of laughter for dinner.

At first, I felt bad about yelling back at the captain because, regardless of the situation, he was my superior. But, as it turned out, he told me that he enjoyed the yelling. To him, all of this was just banter. In the end, we became one big, happy, dysfunctional family.

When there was no shouting, I did a great deal of introspection during the long stretches of manual labor. While sanding and treating wood planks for hours and days on end, with nothing else to do, my mind wandered. Looking around, I found meaning in the situation despite all the challenges it contained. Plus, I felt a deep appreciation for the physical beauty of the world around me. The area across the water from the marina was an old part of town, full of centuries-old buildings featuring unique designs. Looking the other direction, hills rose and fell. *Enchantingly beautiful.*

My mind continuously drifted to the concept of the world around me being a mirror of the world within me. Despite the hurdles I faced, I still found myself in a lovely place, and I wondered what the universe was trying to show me about myself, giving me this yacht reconstruction to work on now. What else within me needed some reconstructing? I would find out soon enough, discovering significant parts of myself in need of repair and renovation that, like this boat, I had no skills to manage.

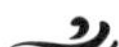

I learned a lot while restoring that old boat in Croatia. I developed new skills, not just in terms of carpentry and mechanics but also in terms of how to work with challenging people such as the captain. One of the biggest lessons lay in how, finally, I realized that when the captain was yelling at or using harsh language toward me, he wasn't trying to harm me. He spoke that way to everybody. This was just how he did things. He was just being himself. Perhaps his manner of communication wasn't what I was used to or even what I preferred, but once I recognized that none of that had anything to do with me, I stopped finding anything offensive about it.

That said, sometimes, I needed to blow off some steam.

As my regular escape from the boat, I'd spend an hour or two at a local gym in town every day. This gym had the absolute bare essentials, an old-school iron paradise full of weights and barbells and equipment that had to be twenty or thirty years old. I quickly fell in love with it. The owner and I became friends. He would share training tips in his broken English, and I would train with locals who spoke zero English. I found it remarkable the way that you don't even need to speak someone's language to successfully accomplish a common goal with them. Those daily gym sessions became a source of sanity, and taking care of my body gave me a way to also take care of my mind.

At day's end, I'd sit on the boat to watch the sun set behind the hills and throw its colors across the Adriatic Sea. Those moments never failed to evoke a sense of awe. *I am really lucky,* I would think.

Those spots of solitary reflection refreshed me and had a way of helping me sleep well so I'd wake up the next morning somehow energized to endure the grind of the workday all over again. They reminded me that, no matter the hardships I faced, life also always offered moments of peace and beauty for me to find. Maybe I was a world away from friends and family, but these sunsets were beautiful, and that was the same sun I'd known all twenty-seven years of my life.

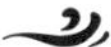

While working aboard the boat in Croatia one day, I saw the first trailer for my season of *Below Deck* released on social media. My life began to noticeably change from that point forward. The captain, stewardess, and chef working on this boat were all fans of the show, as it turned out. So, of course, they immediately recognized me and started having some fun with that, giving me shit for being a celebrity and calling me a bigshot and other silly things.

Then, as more trailers and promotional materials came out over the coming weeks and months, my follower counts began to skyrocket on social media, particularly on Instagram. I started receiving dozens of random direct messages from people I'd never met in my life. By this point, of course, I knew that the show had a large and dedicated fanbase, but still, somehow, it never crossed my mind the way that this could end up affecting me directly. Of course, at this point, it seemed obvious, and I felt a little foolish for not thinking through exactly how things would play out, particularly on social media.

*Holy shit,* I thought. *This might become kind of a big deal.*

I felt grateful to be on my little old boat when all of this started up. What was happening with *Below Deck* couldn't take up so much of my mind when I had a yacht to get ready for going out to sea. The manual labor became another sort of escape for me. I had to make sure this watercraft was ready to give guests a proper yachting experience without somebody getting hurt or, you know, the boat sinking to the bottom of the ocean. These would be simple milk runs throughout the Adriatic, but even still, the sea can be a fickle mistress, and we needed to be prepared for everything.

Miraculously, we did meet our deadline of becoming seaworthy within a month's time, but as we began embarking on charters, something would go wrong with every outing. On one charter, the air conditioning broke. On another, the water pump failed. Meanwhile, the captain's communication style became a bit of an issue with the guests, some of whom had a hard time interacting with him. Others could barely even understand what he was saying. I found myself acting as an interpreter and intermediary between the captain and the guests, attempting to keep the guests feeling safe and excited about being aboard while also helping the captain feel calm and confident in what we were doing.

After a few months, I also began to help with piloting the yacht once we were out to sea. The captain taught me how to do various maneuvers, use the navigational tools, read charts, and manage various other duties associated with being a captain.

One night, while watching the captain navigate in the pitch dark, I found myself mesmerized. We had no way of seeing where we were going, yet he knew exactly where we were and what to do, all simply from the different tools and instruments on the console. Later, that struck me as an interesting metaphor. I might not always be able to see exactly where I was going in life, but there were tools and instruments at my disposal that could still guide my way.

Later, when the yacht's owner learned that I was interested in all that, he allowed me to fly to Turkey for a month to take the necessary classes that would enable me to qualify for a captain's license.

Meanwhile, in Croatia, we began to work better together as a crew. As with all things, the more you do something, the better you get at it. That proved true in this case as well. Charters began to run more smoothly, guests began to have more fun, the captain began to relax more, and our little old boat began to actually behave. Perhaps as a result, guests started leaving larger tips. For a short while, things seemed to be moving in a positive direction.

Alas, such charters proved an inconsistent experience. Our captain and the boat alike were temperamental creatures, and life continued as one big emotional roller coaster. I delighted in the irony of the challenging situation I faced here in Croatia juxtaposed with the minor amount of fame I began to experience, even though my season of the show still had yet to air. Guests consistently began to recognize me from the *Below Deck* promotions, taking selfies with me, telling me how excited they were to meet me and how much they were looking forward to the show.

This ironic situation was sometimes tough to manage. On one hand, I was a budding minor celebrity on television and social media; on the other hand, I felt deep in the trenches on one of the most difficult jobs I'd ever worked in my life, serving a captain who constantly cursed me out aboard a yacht that daily fell apart. No matter how positive and understanding I tried to remain, the circumstances wore on me.

After these long days full of manual and emotional labor, I'd enter my closet of a room and collapse into my tiny bunk, exhausted and laughing at my life. Don't get me wrong—I adored the contradictory experiences. I felt like I was exactly where I was supposed to be, both physically and emotionally. I enjoyed the pseudo-celebrity side of what was starting to happen in my life, and I equally enjoyed the challenge I faced here in Croatia.

The incredible balance was not lost on me as I again recalled the lessons I'd learned from Dr. DeMartini and that TAG workshop, which now felt like ages ago. All of life comes with balance. In Tahiti, working a luxury superyacht on a reality television show, I'd nearly lost my life. Now, as that experience began to bring me fame and—I hoped—better opportunities on the other side, I found myself here in this small boat, doing extremely hard work, feeling more or less alone.

Having gotten a taste of the entertainment industry and its ample bullshit, I reveled in the humility my current situation forced upon me. When I'd started this journey two years prior, I'd never aspired to any sort of fame, never feeling drawn to the vapid nature of the celebrity industrial complex. I'd started this journey in search of fulfillment, true joy, and authentic peace in a world that felt more confusing the more I grew up. This job was perfect for reminding me to always keep my mindset right here. No matter what sort of fame or drama might follow the airing of *Below Deck,* I was prompted to remain humble and reflective, always focused on growth and serving others.

I wanted to develop as a human being and explore the world in a way that paid my bills while allowing me to make other people happy. I was doing exactly that, whether on reality television as a pseudo-celebrity or on a ragtag crew aboard a charmingly decrepit yacht in Croatia. So, regardless of the ups and downs of my experience on this little boat, I was happy.

This was life with two feet in the yachting boat, alright. And just like for anyone in a boat at sea, life was full of beauty and storms.

# CHAPTER 18

After several months aboard the yacht in Croatia, charter season was coming to a close, and the owner offered me a reprieve. Yacht crew members commonly find themselves asked to tend to their yacht owners' homes and other affairs off boat, and likewise, the owner asked me to help with some matters at his house. Knowing my passion for fitness, he first wanted me to help him build a home gym. While we developed that, he also wanted me to tend to other needs around his property.

For the next couple of months, I lived and worked in his 22,000-square-foot mansion. My days began by waking up at the same time as him and his wife and giving them a training session for one to two hours. Then, I'd spend the rest of the workday developing their home gym and taking care of anything else that I could help them with around the grounds.

Soon, I realized my job was essentially to serve as a house boy. I hung holiday decorations, drove the wife around the city in the family's Rolls Royce, helped the husband fix various things around the home, babysat the kids, and so on. Although this felt a bit odd to me, I embraced the opportunity and saw this as a chance to learn from him and his family. They were massively wealthy, their marriage seemed strong, and they seemed to have good relationships with their children.

Even still, while I won't divulge any details out of respect for the family, I saw that they had their share of problems as well. I valued the insight this provided me, as I learned something firsthand that we all have to learn someday: The old cliché is true that money does not bring you total happiness. No matter how much money we have or what sort of lifestyle we lead, all our lives come with their own forms of stress and their own sources of worry. In this family's case, their problems were simply more expensive than mine—sometimes, *much* more expensive. I felt grateful for this opportunity to learn that lesson in a tangible way.

As I worked for this family, my experience with them showed me that while, of course, I wanted to make as much money as I could, money wasn't as important to me as I'd once thought. They were extremely wealthy, but they still had problems, just like anybody. This helped to confirm for me a theory I'd been considering about life: You will always have problems, and you just need to consider which problems are better to deal with than others. I realized that we can't avoid problems, regardless of our circumstances. Different people just have different issues that they're dealing with.

Overall, this was a great perspective for me at this very transitional time in my life. I felt like living with this family gave me a glimpse into what goes into living this type of lifestyle. I have always been ambitious, so I felt like I had this experience for a reason.

As my season of *Below Deck* began to air, the repercussions of being on reality television finally sank in. That hadn't *just* been another interesting, new experience aboard a yacht. It was also something that tons of people were watching. People knew who I was now. Of course, I'd always understood that on a conceptual level, but now, I was actually living that reality.

I found this . . . terrifying. Remember, I'm a shy person by nature. Sure, seeing myself on television, watching the show unfold—all of that felt exciting. However, as part of that, other people were also seeing me and getting to know that version of me. I felt as though a portal had been opened that allowed people access to me and my life in a sense. One million people per week were now watching a show on which I was a prominent member, on full display. They had *opinions* about *me.*

For instance, in the episode showing our first night out at the bar, when I had drunkenly argued with the others about returning to the yacht earlier than I wanted to, I came off a bit like a jackass on television. Seeing that made me laugh, though, because I knew that the crew and I had had a good time that night. Having lived it, I was aware that this was, ultimately, a harmless and funny case of a guy who got drunk and simply didn't want the good time to end. (This happened to me often by the way.)

Then, the show arrived at the episode where I nearly died. At first, I felt shaken up all over again as I relived the incident. However, this showed me that I had apparently done the necessary work to heal from the trauma of that event. My time spent on manual labor and all the other experiences here in Croatia had helped me to heal and move past all of the pain and fear that had imprinted itself in my body.

Plus, for the first time, I witnessed this from an outsider's perspective and saw the outstanding heroism of the cameraman who'd untied the line to save me as well as how concerned the rest of the cast and crew had been for me. I also found meaning and affirmation in the way the crew rallied around me in the aftermath, especially as I recalled how much more had occurred behind the scenes as everyone made sure that I was okay.

In a way, this even made me feel proud of myself. I realized how significant it was that I was able to witness myself living through such a traumatic event and carry myself with more poise and grace than I thought that I had—certainly with more than I was feeling, emotionally, at the time.

Then, there was the love I received on social media. That episode resonated with countless people, and I couldn't keep up with all the messages I received. Strangers all around the world were reaching out to me to tell me that they were happy that I was alive and well.

Perhaps more than anything else so far, this once again gave me that sense of awe and gratitude that just made me think, *What has my life become?*

At one point during the season, the show's producers had me fly back to America to appear on *Watch What Happens Live* with Andy Cohen. Yet again, they booked me a flight and had a driver greet me at the airport and drive me to my hotel. Only this time, we were not in Los Angeles but rather New York City—another incredible new place to explore.

Walking the streets of New York, I felt as though I had stepped into a movie scene. The energy of the city overwhelmed me—yellow taxis flying every direction, steam and smoke filling the air, and people swarming all over the streets, all of it a sea of endless hustle and bustle and noise. I experienced complete and total sensory overload. Being there as a single individual amidst the crowds and buildings and perpetual chaos made me feel irrelevant against the enormity of everything around me. Yet, at the same time, I also felt a spark of infinite possibility. I was struck by a sense that many people experience upon stepping foot in New York City: *Anything can happen.* I loved being there.

New York offered so much more to do than where I'd stayed in L.A. I would hang out at the hotel bar for a bit, go somewhere nice for dinner, then hit a club or two. As all of this was going on, to my complete shock, strangers walking past me on the sidewalk often recognized me from the show and asked to take pictures with me. For some reason, I felt embarrassed and humbled but also deeply flattered. Mostly, this triggered a feeling of complete disbelief.

During Andy's show, I kept thinking about my journey to this point. Not too long ago, I had just been some guy in South Africa who wanted to work on boats. Now, I'd become a recognizable member of a television show, for which I'd been flown to New York City. Now, people recognized me as I walked the streets, and I was being interviewed about all of this on another television show.

*Insane,* was all I kept thinking. *This is all just insane.*

With no idea what waited for me next, I kept checking in with myself, reminding myself to never let any of this get to my head. I wanted to simply stay in the moment and enjoy all of this because it would probably never happen again. A wide range of emotions kept rising and falling within me, and questions cycled with them: *What would this lead to? Could I continue to improve in a way that would eventually top this experience? Would I make something more of myself? Do I even deserve this? Don't they all know I'm just some bro from JoBurg?*

As I finished that trip and returned to Croatia while the rest of the season played out, I refocused on my mantra. *Security in the unknown.* I had no way of knowing any of the answers to those questions. Anything was possible. All I could do was surrender to the experience happening right now, have fun with the interview and with the strangers who suddenly knew me, and remember to be my free-spirited, happy-go-lucky self. Reconnecting with that, I found peace and joy again and decided that I would make the best of whatever came next, no matter what it was.

I had no idea that a fantastic opportunity was right around the corner. By the end of the season, the producers asked me to come back for a second season on the show. This time, they were going to Thailand. Without hesitation, I said yes.

# CHAPTER 19

After spending another month or so working in my Croatian yacht boss's house, I returned home to South Africa and began making preparations for my next season on *Below Deck.* During that period of waiting, I began to notice more oddities about life as a person with some manner of celebrity status.

One of the primary things I observed was how people around me assumed that I was rich now. In their eyes, I had some fame, I had a lot of people following me on social media, and I was about to go shoot another season of this show. None of this translated directly to unusually large income, however. Remember, my first season of *Below Deck* had paid me around the same as I would've been paid to work on any other luxury yacht during that same period. Granted, for my second season, I would earn more, which I looked forward to. Even still, that wasn't going to make me rich.

That said, this would present me with a unique opportunity that I hoped to leverage in a positive manner. Although the pay itself wouldn't make me rich, the following that *Below Deck* offered me through social media could be an excellent asset for the right entrepreneurial idea. The more I learned about the show and reality television in general, the more I realized that cast members often take their newfound visibility and parlay that into a successful business venture.

As a fitness enthusiast, I began to consider the possibilities for building an online coaching business of sorts when the time was right. That could be a unique means by which to continue creating a life for myself that I loved—and to truly help others at the same time. I presented myself with that challenge: With this new fame and the following it provided for me, what good could I do with it?

Although I maintained that open mindset, I felt no hurry to begin a different career. I loved yachting, and now that I had a bit more experience under my belt, both as a yachtie and a reality television cast member, I was looking forward to the new season of *Below Deck.*

Little did I know that this would be the last season I would ever shoot for them. Once again, I would find myself stepping into the wrong place at the wrong time and, thus, hurled into the sea, wrapped in a line threatening to tear me apart. This time, that would happen in a figurative sense, but it would be just as damaging and painful.

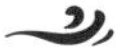

The new season of *Below Deck* began in similar fashion to my first as I was flown to Phuket, Thailand; chauffeured to a hotel; and hustled to my room in secret. Our yacht was docked on the eastern side of Phuket Island at Ao Po Grand Marina, near where Phang Nga Bay meets the Andaman Sea. The surrounding areas offered ample opportunity for breathtaking experiences that we could give our guests, and our home port was situated in a popular area full of wonderful restaurants, bars, and clubs.

While I felt some butterflies in anticipation of meeting my new crew and acclimating to the cameras again, this time, I felt none of the raw nerves that I had experienced before season one. Now, I actually felt like I knew just what I was getting into. I was relaxed and confident and excited, and I felt prepared to have a great season with the show.

While I was eager to participate in my second season of *Below Deck*, I did experience some apprehension in response to the last-minute decision to make me the bosun this time around. Being a bosun means essentially running the ship for Captain Lee, making sure all the crew members handle their duties, doing plenty of work yourself, and maintaining a stoic, respectful demeanor the entire time. To do all of that for the first time on any superyacht would be incredibly stressful. To do all of that for the first time on a superyacht with a whole reality television crew following your every move? With cameras in every corner of the boat?

Since Chandler had struggled the year before, I also felt this sense of pressure to make sure that, if I somehow really *was* the bosun, I would show up in a bigger and better way and do a brilliant job. In no way did I feel up to that task. I did not feel like I was the right man for the job. Last season had been onerous enough, and I'd spent half of it as a junior deckhand and the other half as mere lead deckhand. Becoming a bosun would be a full-blown leadership role for which I knew I was nowhere near prepared. Surely, they must have made some mistake.

The next day, the day we were due to start filming, the producer reassured me that they all believed in me, they knew that I could handle the job, and they were looking forward to this season with me in that position. While that felt like a nice compliment, it did little to extinguish my anxiety. If anything, it might have made it worse because those were all just more expectations that I had to live up to.

Of course, I'd never backed down from a challenge in my life, and once again, I faced a challenge that I had every intention of facing head on, same as always. Just *holy shit*, man. Yet again, I found myself wondering, *How did I get myself into THIS now?*

As the producer walked me out of the hotel and through the Phuket streets toward the marina, I allowed myself to feel every wave of emotion that passed over me. Things felt pretty real for me at this point. I kept thinking about how I'd never been bosun on a boat and recollected all the tension and controversy I'd witnessed between Chandler and Rhylee, then Rhylee and Ross. I asked the producer if she could tell me who the other crew members would be—the more familiar faces, the better—but other than confirming Captain Lee and chief stew Kate, who'd already been announced, the producer told me that she had to keep the cast secret.

As I allowed the apprehension to wash over me, I reconnected with my inner confidence as well. As usual, I dwelled upon my mantra—*security in the unknown*—and reminded myself that this was just my next challenge. Nothing in my life ever went how I expected it to go anyway, so why should I be surprised that this experience was starting off any different?

As we approached the yacht, I saw the camera crew aboard and felt that now familiar sense of not just boarding a yacht but also walking onto a television set. The first person I met on board was Captain Lee. Seeing him again felt great, and as we talked about my new role as bosun and all the anxiety I felt about it, he reassured me that he had total confidence in me, which did infuse me with some sense of calm.

Reconnecting with Kate helped center me as well. Not only was she a familiar face, but having her as chief stew on the interior provided additional reassurance because we'd gotten along well during the previous season. I'd always felt a sense of connection with her, and I never had the slightest doubt that she was great at her job. I knew that she would take care of business on her end, and I felt grateful to have her there.

Other than that, the rest of the cast and crew were all new faces. One of my deckhands, Brian, was a fellow South African. The other two members of the deck crew, Tanner and Abby, both came with sufficient experience under their belts, indicating proper work ethic, and they had great attitudes.

As our charters began, I made my priority maintaining a positive vibe on board, ensuring everyone had a clear sense of their duties every day and providing everyone as much support as they needed to feel confident in handling their responsibilities. All three of my deckhands proved to be excellent workers, and despite feeling overwhelmed at times in this new position as bosun, I felt as though, by and large, everything was going well. We experienced little drama, the guests generally seemed happy and well taken care of, and other than the standard deck crew work stress, I felt that things were going as smoothly as could be expected.

The only hiccup was Abby having an increasingly difficult time with all the cameras. By nature, she had a relaxed, cool demeanor. She could easily just go with the flow, and she always completed any work given to her. However, constantly being on film started to wear on her nerves. In addition, she was in love with a man working on another boat elsewhere in the world, so she started to have a lot of emotions about that. Then, he proposed to her one night, right over the phone. After that, Abby just needed to go be with him, so she resigned from her post and left the yacht.

I was disappointed to see her go because she had been a great crew member with an outstanding disposition, which my growing experience had started to show me was invaluable. Still, I understood. Love is love. I felt happy for her that she had found someone to marry and spend her life with. Anyway, who could possibly begrudge someone leaving a reality television show to go be with the one they love?

My primary concern was that whoever replaced Abby be just as strong of a worker with an equally positive attitude. I'd settled into a nice rhythm with the crew, our camaraderie and chemistry had been working well, and we all felt we understood each other. Although I had no say in who Captain Lee and the producers hired as Abby's replacement, I hoped they would find someone similar to her so that we could finish the season without drama or unnecessary stress.

When Captain Lee called me up to the wheelhouse to talk about Abby's replacement, he said that he'd made a decision, so I asked him if he had a CV that I could review. He said I wouldn't need one because I already knew them. With a funny little smile on his face, Captain Lee told me that he had hired Rhylee.

Although I naturally felt a bit of anxiety as I remembered how things had gone between Rhylee and the crew the previous season, my focus immediately went to what I could do to create as many good vibes with her as possible. I chose to believe the best and was determined to do whatever I needed to do to maintain a harmonious environment within my crew. Clearly, Rhylee felt sensitive to being disrespected even where disrespect wasn't intended, so I wanted to be cognizant of that and sensitive toward her in kind. My goal became to keep her feeling included and safe and supported and give her as much opportunity to grow as possible.

When she came aboard, I gave her a warm greeting, and after she met with Captain Lee and settled into her bunk, I caught up with her during a bit of downtime. I pulled her aside and told her I knew the previous season had been a bit rough and that her relationships with the last two bosuns hadn't been the best, but I wanted her to know that I'd give her what she needed to feel supported. We still had a lot of the season ahead of us, and it was important to me that we have a productive season without any of the conflict and controversy that had taken place last year. Whatever had happened previously, I told her that I carried no negative feelings into this season as a result, and I hoped that she felt the same. I felt like she received this well, and we ended on a good note after a healthy conversation, giving me some peace and hope moving forward.

A couple of nights later, after finishing our latest charter, everyone on the crew went to dinner at a restaurant near port. After we all sat down as a big group and perused the menu, we deferred to our chef, Kevin, saying that he should use his expertise to make some selections for the table, and we could all share. That led to a conversation between Kevin and Rhylee that somehow escalated into a shouting match. Everyone else kept quiet, hoping this would die out quickly, but it did not. They kept going until they were so loud that people throughout the restaurant were turning to look, restaurant employees were eyeballing us and talking amongst themselves, and we all started to feel embarrassed.

Along with some of the other members of the crew, I decided to leave the table and walk down toward the beach. Since we were off duty and trying to simply enjoy a nice, relaxing evening off the boat, and since I had determined to let go of any hard feelings that might have been related to the previous season, I preferred to avoid the conflict, believing that Rhylee and Kevin could resolve their issue themselves.

However, the fight moved from the table to the beach. Instead of resolving and fading, it continued to increase in hostility until it reached a boiling point that compelled me and a few others to intervene. When even that failed to settle the situation, I began to grow irritated. At one point, I rolled my eyes and said, “Oh my god. Here we go again. This is just more of the same.”

That led to Rhylee directing some of her vitriol toward me, and then the two of us further exchanged some words. In far too little time, what had started out as a nice dinner had rapidly exploded into this huge shitshow, the likes of which we'd never remotely approached in several prior outings together as a crew. This is just my perspective, but I strongly suspected Rhylee was playing up the drama for the camera.

The truth was that part of me liked Rhylee. I respected her. She had myriad strengths. She was passionate, she had a great work ethic, and she never failed to stand up for what she believed was right. If she thought you had wronged her, she would never keep quiet or back down from you. I could see how, in her personal life, this was a generally positive trait to have.

I decided that if she kept that aggressiveness isolated to her personal life and didn't bring it into her work aboard the yacht itself, then I could deal with her. So, at some point later that evening or the next morning, I approached her, and we talked through the situation as I tried to find common ground with her. We agreed that we just wanted to have a good season the rest of the way and do whatever we could to prevent such conflicts from interfering with the work we needed to do aboard the yacht.

As a bosun in my first managerial position, I had begun to learn a bit about the different archetypes of people in a work environment. In Rhylee's case, she simply fell onto one of the more extreme ends of the spectrum, where she was very outspoken and passionate. I did empathize with her because, clearly, all that built-up anger came from somewhere.

That presented me with a challenge I wanted to manage in a healthy way, not only for me as the bosun but also for everybody else on the boat. I worried about my ability to handle such a strong personality with dramatically limited experience in a managerial position, and I hoped that Rhylee would be able to tell that I held respect for her and only wanted the best for the crew. To my mind, the goal was always to put aside my personal feelings in favor of working together for the greater good of the charter and for the overall success of the yacht.

Unfortunately, that's not how things played out between me and Rhylee. She continued to conduct herself the same way she always had. When given tasks she disliked, she responded with attitude. When her attitude was addressed, instead of understanding the issue, she chose to get defensive and combative, inevitably escalating a minor conflict into a major fight, time after time. Conflicting personalities are unavoidable sometimes, but there are also healthy ways to address that conflict, and none of them involve starting a shouting match in front of the crew.

Once again, the primary issue from my perspective seemed to be Rhylee's inability to respect the hierarchy of being on a crew. As a junior deckhand, you always approach the job with the mentality that whatever the boss says goes.

Remember, for instance, my first job aboard *The Gene Machine.* When I first arrived for day work and realized that they had hired somebody else when I thought they should have hired me, I was furious. However, I kept those emotions to myself, gave the entire crew my best face, and channeled my frustration into my work and into earning the respect that I felt I had been deprived of. Had I handled that situation the way Rhylee handled her feelings here, then I would have been asked to leave the boat on the very first day.

All of that said, I wish I had done a better job engaging with her in a more compassionate manner. Instead, when we did have those conflicts, I allowed myself to get swept up in the emotion of the moment. I frequently became defensive and offended myself, which, in hindsight, also proved unhelpful and unproductive.

I have empathy for myself as I reflect on this because I can see how overwhelmed I was by all my new responsibilities, but I also feel for Rhylee because she clearly wasn't feeling good herself. I can't help but wonder what else I could have done to better foster a healthier emotional environment for her as well. As someone who has also gone through hardship and dealt with many challenges in life, I relate to feeling frustrated, and I feel I could have done a better job *connecting* with Rhylee instead of simply *arguing* with her.

Regardless, no matter how I tried to communicate with Rhylee and improve the health of our working environment, nothing seemed to be working, and everybody seemed to be growing increasingly unhappy. As the season carried on, crew members kept finding themselves engaged in more and more conflict, and tensions continued to escalate as morale deteriorated.

At one point, Brian pulled me aside and expressed to me that he wasn't sure how to continue because he was so tired of Rhylee fighting with him and everyone else. He made an offhand comment saying that he would rather go a man down if that meant not having to deal with Rhylee on board any longer. When he said that, I took notice because if he felt that strongly about how detrimental the environment had become, then that was a serious matter. While I wasn't certain about outright having Rhylee removed from the crew, I understood Brian's perspective.

Before engaging with Rhylee about this or taking it to Captain Lee, I wanted to see what Tanner thought since he was the other member of the deck crew. Now, Tanner and I had had our fair share of disagreements as well. However, Tanner seemed to take direction and respond to criticism better than Rhylee, and it was important to me to consider his perspective despite any conflict we may have had in the past. After all, as the leader, I wanted to understand what everyone was feeling. Unfortunately, when I spoke with Tanner and shared Brian's feelings with him, Tanner said that he felt the same way.

At this point, I realized one of the primary problems: There was no more joy in this job. All of us were miserable. Everyone was fighting. Finding ourselves in a situation like this went against everything that had drawn us to this industry in the first place. We were here to work hard, yes, but we were also here to enjoy our lives, explore new things, and have fun while we did it. With everything going on, none of that was happening.

Now that I knew three out of the four members of the deck crew, including me, felt the same way due to the fourth crew member, I contemplated my next steps as a leader in this situation. What needed to happen now? I was tempted to commiserate with Tanner and Brian—to simply say, "Yes, this sucks, but if we put our minds to it, we can endure the situation until the season is over and just try to avoid conflict as much as possible." In the meantime, I could also talk to Rhylee about how everyone was feeling, trust her not to explode over that as well, and hope that her behavior would improve. I wondered if that would be the healthiest and most peaceful solution, but I also had serious doubts as to whether that would be sustainable. We all felt like we were walking on eggshells already and were absolutely exhausted as a result.

I contemplated what other actions I could take to defuse tensions and starve the drama. Maybe I could do more to accommodate Rhylee and make her feel more comfortable. Clearly, she had a problem with feeling threatened. Any perceived insult or disrespect, true or not from my perspective, felt true and painful to her, and she had to fight against it. Similar to the captain in Croatia, her difficult temperament had nothing to do with me. I had to remember that. In response, I could work harder to stop allowing myself to get caught up in the behavior and to maintain a more mature and sound perspective. Now, in hindsight, I wish I'd had the tools and the ability to help myself—and my other crew members—respond in a more productive way. We didn't *have* to have a reaction to her at all times.

However, I also kept thinking to myself that perhaps this was an opportunity for me to stand up for what I believed in. I considered what would happen on other boats if this situation arose. How would other leaders I'd worked for respond if faced with this kind of behavior? Did I feel that they would ask three of their four deck crew members to bear the weight of the fourth's bad attitude—or would they do something about the fourth, whose personality and choices consistently created and escalated conflict?

Something else that kept going through my mind was Ross during the previous season when he'd said that he should have just fired Rhylee when he had the chance. I now felt like I was in a similar position as he had been.

I knew that Rhylee had many strengths and much to offer—there was a reason that she was here, after all—and I desperately wanted to find a diplomatic solution that kept her aboard while also creating a healthy work environment again. So, I kept thinking about going to her and talking things through. But then I kept remembering all the previous times I had done so and how unfruitful those efforts had been. In addition, I felt that if I continued in that vein, not only was I beating my head against a figurative wall, but I was also taking the easy way out as a leader. It made it seem like I was afraid to make a bigger, much more difficult choice.

As I went back and forth in my own mind, I considered discussing this with Captain Lee multiple times, but I always stopped myself from doing so. Captain Lee often made clear points that he didn't need to be bothered by such petty matters on the boat. He liked to say that he had leaders to handle such things for him and that we were responsible for making the choices necessary for the good of our crew.

After much contemplation, I felt that I needed to be the person who could make difficult decisions, even if they might somehow reflect badly on me. It was the right thing to do if I believed those tough calls would ultimately be in the best interest of the crew and the yacht as a whole. I needed to ask Captain Lee to fire Rhylee from the crew, same as he had Chandler the season before.

This terrified me. However, it was what my gut told me was the right move at this moment, and as scared as I felt, I also believed that Captain Lee would respect this decision and the reasoning behind it. I had been selected as bosun for a reason, and this felt like one of those moments when I had to rise to the level of my responsibilities.

Working up the nerve to approach Captain Lee about this took some time. When I finally found the courage, I approached him during a quiet afternoon in the bridge deck aft, which had become his quarters for a charter as he'd offered his room to another guest. When I laid the situation out for him, he seemed to understand and respect me coming to him with my concerns. At the time, he told me that he would think about it and get back to me. Then, later, he called me back to tell me that he disagreed with my decision and that we would not be removing Rhylee from the crew.

I left that conversation feeling stung, small, confused, and insecure. Unsure of how to process his response, I fell deep into a mindset of completely doubting myself. I second-guessed everything that had led up to my decision and contemplated every possible way I could have been wrong. *What have I missed? What did I fail to consider? Did I make the wrong choice? Have I not actually thought this through correctly? Was everything I had learned on previous boats not the right way to manage and live within a crew?*

I kept replaying something Captain Lee had said to me: "You don't just get rid of someone."

Maybe I'd done a poor job communicating with him? Later, he said that I had only focused on Rhylee's flaws, not enough on her strengths, and that when we have problems with someone on the crew, we work them out instead of simply kicking them to the curb. In my mind, I *had* focused a great deal on Rhylee's strengths, and I *had* tried working things out with her for a long time before even considering this drastic course of action.

This wasn't a decision I had just made on an impulse. There had been a long buildup to this. We'd gone through one whole season with her behaving this way. We'd taken a lot of shit from her back then. When she came back, I'd tried to talk with her and create a healthy environment for her and everyone else. I'd done my best to deal with each issue through conversation and compromise and finding mutual understanding. I'd put in a lot of effort. Surely, I thought, a captain would respect his bosun having to arrive at this sort of decision.

But then, later on, I heard that Captain Lee's reasoning to deny my request was based in large part on the fact that Kate, our chief stew, had also approached him about Rhylee and given him an argument for why she *shouldn't* be fired.

When I heard that, my head really started to spin. I worked with Rhylee all day, every day, while Kate spent possibly 10 percent of her time on the boat involved with anything related to the deck crew, let alone Rhylee. All Kate knew, as Rhylee's bunkmate, was what Rhylee told her at the end of each day, and I doubted that Rhylee was providing the most unbiased account of events. Yet Kate had become the deciding factor in Rhylee remaining on board—not the bosun of the yacht, who had been enduring Rhylee's volatility all this time.

Feeling defeated, my self-confidence dropped to zero, and I questioned everything about myself. I felt as though I no longer understood anything about management, running a yacht, or even life itself.

There was no choice at that point but to accept the situation and move forward. I resolved to simply do the best I could with the situation at hand and, along the way, have as much fun as possible. In my case, that also meant leaning hard into my passion for partying. I began to drink harder and harder on our nights out on the town, and as that continued throughout the latter part of the season, I found myself making that figurative misstep that would go on to tear me apart.

# CHAPTER 20

The *Below Deck* family had come to know and love Smashton dating back to my first season on the show, and as the stresses of my second season compounded, Smashton began to show up more frequently and with growing intensity. I engaged in my fair share of drunken foolishness during my Smashton nights and had to make more apologies than I felt proud of. For the most part, however, that had all been the good side of Smashton—the carefree, fun-loving version of myself that I still secretly hoped to get more in touch with while sober.

Unfortunately, as I mentioned previously, Smashton had a dark side that would make an appearance once or twice a year, and during an especially drunken evening following one of our later charters, he came out and did some real damage.

It occurred during a night of drinking to the point of obliteration. I actually didn't even realize exactly what I did until I saw the footage months later. All I recalled was a hazy, emotional cab ride back to the yacht, during which Kate and I apparently found ourselves in a heated argument.

The next morning, Kate was gone from the yacht, and I was struggling to understand what had happened the night before. When Kate hadn't returned in time to begin our work shift that morning, I went to Captain Lee and explained to him what had happened to the best of my memory, saying that during our night out, Kate and I had had an argument, and I thought that was why she was gone. Nobody else seemed to remember much either, only telling me that she and I had exchanged some harsh words. So, nobody divulged the finer details of what took place.

I felt horrible. Kate had never been one of my closest friends, but I'd always liked her. In fact, we'd stayed in touch a bit between seasons, and she'd given me some good advice as a veteran of the show. We didn't agree on everything, but I appreciated her. I thought she was a good person, and her immense value to the yacht and the show went without saying. This season, however, we did have our fair share of butting heads.

Thankfully, Kate returned later that morning. When we spoke, I told her that I didn't really remember what had happened, but I'd obviously been a jackass. With utmost sincerity, I said I felt bad about everything and apologized. Then, I was sure to make clear that I respected her, our relationship meant a lot to me, and I hoped things would be okay with us moving forward. She gave me the impression that she accepted my apology and we could just move on. From there, we never spoke about that night again, and neither did anybody else in the cast.

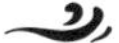

After the season finished filming, Ross invited me to come crash with him on the west coast of Florida in the United States, where he was working on a yacht. He and I had been speaking often, and after the chaos of the season, I needed some time with a good friend who would understand what I'd gone through and who allowed me to simply be myself. For a few weeks, I stayed at his place, relaxed, unwound, living off the cash from *Below Deck.* I regularly let Smashton out, partying hard with Ross.

From there, I visited another friend on Florida's east coast, and while there, I connected with a boat captain who offered me a job on a small yacht based out of St. Petersburg. The boat was smaller than I'd worked on before and had a small crew that consisted of the captain, me, and a stewardess who doubled as a chef. We served a lovely couple with four kids and their friends, making trips with them to the Bahamas and throughout the Caribbean. For various legs of the journeys, the captain allowed me to put my captain's license to use myself and do some navigating and docking. Having been a captain for many years, he taught me a great deal more about the craft. The entire experience was fulfilling, reminding me once again why I'd pursued a career in this industry in the first place.

Upon returning to St. Petersburg, I began dating a wonderful woman and enjoyed my time with her while resting some more and trying to decide my next career move. As I waited for my season of *Below Deck* to air, I also wanted to wait and see if the producers would ask me back for a third season.

A few weeks before the season was scheduled to air, producers again flew me to Los Angeles for a round of pick-up interviews. While I was there, they took me through footage they planned to air, which included a significant amount of time from nights that had been rather hazy in my memory. They had captured Smashton in all his glory. I just sort of laughed my way through it for the interviews, keeping things light and keeping some of my more personal thoughts on the footage to myself.

Then, they showed me footage from the night of my fight with Kate, and what I saw scared me and broke my heart.

After we had all stumbled into the taxi van, having drunk ourselves into oblivion, Tanner, Kevin, and I were joking around. Kate, sitting behind me in the van, said something to me that triggered me . . . I made every effort to turn and face Kate to confront her, but Kevin prevented me from doing so, which prompted a struggle between me and him.

In that moment, during this interview, I got to witness what the built-up anger and aggression I had in me actually looked like . . . Clearly enraged by the situation and reaching the point of absolute frustration, I balled my fist and hammered it into the van window beside me.

During my pick-up interviews, all I could say was that I was shocked at my behavior, I had a hard time accepting the person in that footage, and I felt absolutely terrible about it. As I left Los Angeles, I fell into a somber mood, anticipating the fallout that would come from a million people watching me behave in such a fashion.

Even worse, I couldn't stop thinking about the footage that had opened my eyes to the truth. It was one thing to feel that anger on the inside. Now that I had actually seen it from the outside, I knew that something had to change.

# CHAPTER 21

Upon returning to Florida, I began slipping into something of a depressive state in anticipation of the new season of *Below Deck* hitting the air. When episodes started to come out, my depression deepened. The thoughts I'd kept to myself during the pick-up interviews revolved around the simple fact that, as I watched myself, I didn't know how I felt about the guy I was viewing. As I observed myself going full Smashton and getting so drunk, I no longer saw someone who was having fun. I saw a person who was hurting. Yes, the season had been stressful. I had been facing some challenges the likes of which I'd never faced before, particularly taking on the responsibilities of being a bosun on such short notice and then feeling so lost as far as how to be a proper leader for a personality such as Rhylee.

Even still, as I continued to think about what I had just watched, I mentally took a step back and viewed myself as someone I didn't know. When I did that, I could see that, clearly, this person was dealing with a lot more than simply the stress of the season. He seemed to have pain that ran deep and that he perhaps wasn't even consciously aware of. The person I saw on the screen seemed like somebody who had shit to deal with—shit that he had been neglecting throughout his life.

The more I watched myself drink and party, the more I started noticing red flags about myself. I looked like someone afraid to deal with his life in a sober state of mind, and it seemed I needed alcohol to break free from that fear. As I allowed myself to think my way through these things, I realized that partying and drinking had become my way of coping with issues, past and present, I felt I had no control over.

I thought about the violent and destructive environment created by my mom and dad when I was young. I reflected on them getting divorced, on having to move schools and houses, on witnessing their various relationships with significant others rise and fall. I pondered over all these other things that had happened throughout my life—hardships I now realized I would just push aside without actually dealing with them.

Growing up, I would simply focus on sports and school and having good times with my friends. As I became an adult and started my career, I graduated to the more mature forms of escapism found in partying and drinking. Now, watching myself on this show, I saw flashes of how much all my traumas and insecurities were raging under the surface and shaping me into this unhappy person.

The drinking and the partying were my ways of distracting myself from that trauma. I put enormous pressure on myself to be strong and just soldier on, but that evidently wasn't working great for me. The power of alcohol is that it gives you a reprieve from stress and other negative feelings—but only to a point. Eventually, it becomes more like gasoline you're pouring on a fire.

With each episode airing, I saw the way that I had to drink to get to that carefree state I wished I could live in while sober. There was no denying I seemed to be drinking as a way to evade or forget something. What that was, I wasn't sure, but obviously, I needed to find out and deal with it. There was no way around it as I saw it in technicolor on the screen: I had a lot of work I needed to do on myself.

Then, there was the footage of me raging at Kate and punching the van window.

When that episode aired, I thought about my dad. That was the exact same behavior I'd seen from him when I was a kid. That's what he'd taught me, though probably not intentionally. If you're angry, hit something—break something. He was never violent toward people. Yes, he'd fought his fair share of fights, but he never became physical or aggressive with a significant other or a friend. He would, however, regularly take his anger out on various walls, doors, and other inanimate objects throughout the house.

This was the first time I'd ever seen myself in that state through somebody else's eyes, and I felt like I was a little kid again, watching my dad losing his temper and expressing his anger physically. I'd become emotional, reached a boiling point, exploded, and punched the window. Then, *boom*—I was free of the emotion.

When I saw that, I considered how that had made me feel as a child, so small and terrified and helpless. Then, I considered how I must have made the others feel in that moment—and that was deeply not okay with me.

Hitting that window had nothing to do with Kate or Kevin or anybody else in that van. Watching the footage, I felt terrible for them because, from their perspective, I appeared threatening and frightening. I knew, though, that the way I'd behaved in that conflict with Kate wasn't really about her, despite how things looked. It was just about my own issues, my baggage, my traumas, and so many things in my life that I hadn't properly dealt with.

I felt ashamed and embarrassed and heartbroken. I wish I could say I was surprised, but that's not true because these sorts of things had happened before. But to actually see it for myself was a completely different experience. This wasn't an incident that had just happened with my close group of friends who could laugh it off, who knew me and knew what I'd been through and knew I never meant anyone any harm.

This had happened with people I'd only known for a few months at most—and now, beyond that, it was being aired to an audience of one million strangers. As bad as I felt for myself, I also felt terrible for Kate and Kevin and everyone else involved with the show.

Flooded with those complex emotions, I recorded an apology that I quickly posted to my social media. Then, I essentially froze in a state of paralysis. I had no idea what the right thing to do was at that point. My world was completely turned over. Aside from feeling deep regret over what had happened, I also felt deep uncertainty. I thought I had done a lot of work on myself, but apparently there was a lot more work to be done.

Exactly how and when and where to go about that, I had no idea. My head had started spinning, and I didn't know how to make it stop. And my quest for self-improvement quickly became even more daunting as I began to experience the onslaught of backlash that came my way as a result of the episode. Ultimately, this would become one of those moments in life that show you what you most need to face about yourself and set you on a righteous path full of pain and growth and, ultimately, healing. I would get there—but not all at once and certainly not right at first.

Within the episode itself, Kate had plenty to say about me that she'd never said to me personally before. Captain Lee said that if he had known the full extent of my explosion in the van that night, he would have had me removed from the yacht immediately—and that I would never be on the show again.

I recognized the damage done by my behavior, and I knew that making any sort of amends was not likely to happen in the immediate future. My red flags were waving in my face bright and clear, and I was finally focused on the emotional trauma and baggage that I was carrying as well as the amount of work I needed to do on it.

This was the hard part. I thought I had done so much work and felt like I had overcome a lot of my issues, but there was clearly so much more that needed to be worked through. But then, this is how we grow. We go through circumstances that finally force us to confront all the shit we've been trying not to look at. Something like this had to happen for me to begin to grow and make some healthier choices for myself and my life. I knew that would also be a long process.

In the meantime, I became sidetracked for a bit by the backlash. My girlfriend at the time and I had been hosting watch parties at our friends' bars and restaurants, but now, I was too embarrassed and depressed to attend. All my mature, contemplative reflection found itself in combat against the less evolved, more emotional parts of myself that wanted to get defensive and point fingers at other people for their role in the situation too.

One of the most challenging aspects to all of this, I quickly discovered, was the dark side of social media. You remember that portal I mentioned the show opening into my personal life a few chapters ago? That was still there, and now it was destroying me.

# CHAPTER 22

People began responding to the episode by flooding my various social media account inboxes, and I quickly found myself overwhelmed by both the volume of messages and the intensity of the emotion they contained. A handful of the messages were frightening and painful, as some people told me that I no longer deserved to live and should go kill myself. Other messages, while containing significant resentment, seemed to be motivated instead by a great deal of pain. People were voicing their anger at me for what I had done—because it reminded them of similar, terrible things that had occurred in their own lives.

I found myself feeling a wide range of emotions in response to these messages. Naturally, they sometimes made me feel defensive and even angry myself. But when I allowed those initial feelings of defensiveness to pass, I saw something else deeper than the surface. I saw people who were hurting, and I saw them associating me with their pain and their trauma. Even though I knew that I'd never felt the desire to physically injure a woman—or anyone for that matter—strangers had no possible way of knowing that about me. If they had experienced any sort of violence or pain that was remotely similar, then of course seeing me behave in such an irate and volatile fashion would remind them of what they had endured.

I felt terrible about that. The world had enough pain and heartache as it was, and part of the reason I'd been drawn to the yachting industry was because of its ability to bring people joy. People who watched this show watched it for similar reasons. For me to behave in a way that brought up viewers' worst memories created the antithesis of joy.

At least, that's how I was able to respond *sometimes*. Other times, I became so completely overwhelmed by the flood of messages and the fury I experienced online that my mind began to fall deeper and deeper into a depressive state. Despite empathizing with where many of those messages came from and what motivated the people sending them, I couldn't help but be terribly disturbed by them.

I could tell myself the same things that my friends tried to tell me: *Just ignore it. Don't let it get to you. You made a mistake, but you're trying to learn from it and grow from it, and these people don't know who you really are*. But no matter what, sometimes, I couldn't help but open my inbox, scroll through those messages, and feel like I was emotionally bleeding out over just how hateful some people could be.

The life I'd worked so hard to build for myself now crumbled down all around me, and I found myself second-guessing everything about myself as a human being. *Was I a good person? Was I smart enough to discover exactly how to work on myself? If so, was I strong enough to actually do that work—to see it through?*

The path ahead of me seemed more obscure and uncertain than ever before, and I felt as though I faced a tremendous amount of work along that path. Even if I did do the necessary work on myself, and even if I did heal and grow into a more evolved human being who had truly learned from his mistakes, it wouldn't necessarily make a difference. Everything lives forever on the internet now. Cancel culture had taken hold, and I felt as though people would never see me as anything other than a raging, dangerous asshole, no matter what else I did for the rest of my life, regardless of how sincere I was in my desire to improve myself.

I felt as though no matter who I decided to become next, there would always be people determined to punish me for who I used to be. Any mistakes I'd made would haunt me for the rest of my life.

Perhaps worst of all, I was worried that whenever people recognized me, they would always associate me with their worst feelings and experiences when all I'd ever wanted was to give people joy and laughter and happiness.

I spiraled through these emotions for a few dark, hard months. Shame took firm hold of my heart, and loneliness gripped me in equal measure. Life took on a hollow feeling as though it was suddenly devoid of true substance—empty. Looking at the road I faced ahead, unsure of how to move past the moment I found myself in now, I wasn't certain I even wanted to keep going. I wasn't sure that life was even worth living anymore. As I continued to spiral, thoughts of ending my life began to plague my mind. That terrified me, and yet I couldn't stop thinking about it.

The biggest problem here was that everything those people were saying to me . . . I was also saying to myself. My own biggest critic, I felt as upset with myself as anyone else who cursed me out or told me to kill myself. I had created this situation, after all. Their words hurt because I believed them.

For the first time in my life, I understood why people commit suicide.

Of course, I knew all about mental health as all my decisions that had led me to starting my yachting journey had been based around creating my healthiest state of being. Unfortunately, it's often too late when you realize you need help. At that point, you may ask yourself,

*Is it easier to just end the struggle?* This is what I was dealing with, and I didn't know how to process it effectively.

The men I grew up with would always say, "Big boys don't cry." Extrapolate that across the sum total of life experience, and the message is: To discuss your emotions is to be weak. The world I grew up in was one in which men were meant to become machines. My great-grandfather was raised that way; he drilled that into his son, who then drilled it into his son, who then drilled it into me. Nobody spoke of trauma or wounds or the healing thereof. If you felt something painful, you did what you had to do to stop feeling it and get on with your life. You had to be "strong."

Now, after a lifetime of that, the pain I'd spent my entire existence avoiding had now incapacitated me.

However, the lessons I learned from Dr. DeMartini once again proved true, as the implicate order of the universe came through with its balancing of negatives with positives. That began with the woman I was dating at the time. Without her, I'm not sure how I would have made it through.

Since I was far from home, I got away with presenting a strong front to most of my friends and family back home. Even Ross was across the state of Florida on the opposite coast, so he wasn't fully aware of my emotional state.

My girlfriend at the time, however, saw my collapse. She provided the support I needed in those early days, simply giving me steady, regular reminders that I should and could keep going. In no uncertain terms, she was my rock at this stage in my life, helping me stop doubting myself so much and convincing me to not give up. "Everybody makes mistakes," she told me, "and everybody has embarrassing moments that simply show them where they still need to grow." Mine just happened to occur on an international television show with an audience of over a million.

During all of this, I continued to go out and drink and party, doing the very thing I knew had caused me so many problems. I was drinking to escape from the realization that I had been drinking to escape from my problems.

Finally, I began to recognize how drinking only seemed to amplify the negatives in my life. The numb fun of a drunken night always gave way to a hangover the next day, most of which would be spent lying around feeling sick and not exactly contemplating the good parts of my life. And now, I was started to experience hangovers that would last up to three, even four, days. I spent much of that time lying on the couch, scrolling through negative messages on my phone, and generally wallowing in both physical and emotional misery.

Thinking this through a bit more, I considered how much money I'd been spending going out and drinking only to get home, pass out, and wake up feeling shitty like this without remembering half of what I'd done while drunk. It became unavoidably clear that most of the problems in my life existed because of behavior that had occurred when I was drunk. I asked myself a very simple question: *What is drinking actually adding to my life?*

Doing the math, I arrived at the sobering conclusion that not only was drinking *not* adding to my life in any obvious, meaningful way, but it was also significantly and unignorably subtracting from my life. Nights out would end up with tabs ranging from a couple hundred dollars to a couple thousand. At some point during those nights, after smashing vodkas and/or tequilas until reaching a certain level of intoxication, there came an inevitable conflict or moment of humiliation. The next morning, recall of such events would be hazy at best while I suffered through yet another hangover.

I continued with the math, and here's where I began to do some real work on myself. I simply started asking myself "Why?" over and over again, not unlike a toddler interrogating their parents. Why was I going out and getting shitfaced? Well, I needed to be in a certain state of mind. Why did I need to be in a certain state of mind? Well, because I wanted to feel more carefree and less worried about things in my life. Why did I need to feel that way? Okay, so why did I . . .

And so on down the rabbit hole.

As I began this process of questioning myself and peeling back my layers, I realized that I had much more work to do on myself than I'd realized. The next bit of math seemed obvious by now: I could do that work better and more efficiently with a healthy body and a clear mind. I wanted to be able to identify the things that needed to change and the ways I needed to go about changing them. I needed to be sharp to do that. The better I felt, the better this process would go, and all that alcohol really did was make me feel like shit.

Having performed this elaborate calculus, on January 6, 2020, I told my girlfriend, "I'm done drinking."

Now, she'd heard this sort of sweeping declaration before when I was in the throes of one of my epic hangovers, so she gave me a cordial, "Okay, that sounds great."

But I insisted. "This time, I'm really done."

Looking me in the eyes, feeling my vibe, she nodded. "You know what? I believe you. And I love that for you."

Soon enough, I was able to see that the rest of my life would not, in fact, be characterized by people hating me. My girlfriend pointed out that I was receiving plenty of supportive messages as well, some from friends and family, others from complete strangers who had become fans. Many of them echoed the same things she had been telling me. In so many ways, this was actually a huge gift. This situation had stripped me down to the bare bones of who I was. It was now forcing me to take an honest look at my life and all the things that made me who I was to that point. Now, I saw the work I had to do next.

For your sake, I'd love to tell you that quitting drinking was all I needed to do, and all my problems began to resolve themselves once I became sober. Unfortunately, the truth is more complicated than that. In all honesty, things actually became a lot harder, and I felt a lot worse for a long time after that. Healing surprised me that way. But this was my new challenge to commit to, the new unknown in which I had to find security. In pursuit of healing, I would allow myself to first be ripped apart. That's how I found what I needed to put myself back together.

And yes, it would take work, but this was all just the start of massaging the trauma out of the wound, same as I'd had to do for my ankle after being nearly ripped apart by the tender line. Just because this current moment of my life was painful didn't mean this would last forever. Our most painful moments often lead to our most beautiful days.

# CHAPTER 23

Big changes in life will be met with great resistance. I thought that I'd keep going out sober, but after one or two nights at my usual club spots, that changed. Completely sober in a venue where I used to go wild and dance like a hooligan, I now found myself simply looking around in awe.

Being surrounded by people getting hammered made me laugh, especially because, after about half an hour, I realized that I simply could not handle this environment sober. Suddenly, a place that had once seemed like my favorite source of fun and entertainment felt boring and aggravating. Never had the music seemed so intense and so loud, and never had trying to hold a conversation with somebody felt so aggressive and impossible all at once. I didn't like it there anymore.

After my second sober club outing, I never went back.

Other nights, I'd go to a bar with friends, socializing and catching up and such. That would last until 9:30 or 10 p.m., around the time everyone else was starting to get nice and buzzed and conversations shifted from talking with each other to yelling at each other. I'd wish everyone a fun night, go home, get in bed, and wake up refreshed the next morning. Then, I'd get a workout in and have a fantastic day, amazed at how much time I'd spent in the past just surviving hangovers.

Now that my life and some of my friendships didn't have going out and getting drunk as their foundation, some of us had less in common than we thought, and some people began to seem less comfortable with me. I wondered if it was because the drunk persona of mine that they'd gotten to know so well no longer existed or maybe because the depth of our friendship hadn't been greater than the beers we'd shared.

Others seemed to become uneasy with me when I did go to the bar with them but not drink, especially after they couldn't convince me to at least have "just one drink, mate." I wondered if my sobriety made them uncomfortable with their own drinking. Perhaps they weren't ready to stop drinking yet because of what that would mean they had to confront in their life. Or maybe I just wasn't as fun sober.

My circles began shifting a bit as I started to avoid people who seemed unhappy with me unless I was who they wanted me to be. I became more guarded about who I spent my time with. In some ways, this was painful because a portion of my friends showed their true colors by fading from my life as I held true to my sobriety. In other ways, however, this was revitalizing because I discovered who really did care about me and support me. The people who really love you want you to do what is best for you.

Before long, my emotional and psychological health made notable improvements. I felt more stable and secure, and I started to simply spend more time with myself so that I could begin the deeper work of unpacking and exploring the roots of my issues.

To do this, I continued to interrogate myself, starting with the incident that had set this entire saga in motion: the explosion in the *Below Deck* van. By now, I'd established that the vast majority of my drunken nights out resulted in good times all around, but there were those one or two incidents every year in which I would simply lose my shit. That, to me, wasn't the root issue though. Nor, I realized, was alcohol. During stretches of my life when I'd chosen to be strict with my diet while in training and such, I'd had no problem going weeks or even months without drinking.

*So*, I asked myself, *why do I like alcohol in the first place? Not because it tastes good—most of it tastes like car fuel. So, why do I drink it? Well, maybe because it relaxes me.*

Okay, now we're getting somewhere.

*Why do I need to feel relaxed? Well, I'm stressed out by work or something else.*

*Okay, why are they stressful? Well, they are challenging me in this way and that way on a daily basis.*

*Okay, why are those things challenging for you? Well, this person has a personality that I don't like dealing with.*

*Okay, why do you not like that personality? Well, because my mom or my dad used to treat me like that.*

Okay, now we're *really* getting somewhere—we are getting to the core of what's actually happening.

During these interrogations, I remembered the simple fact that I am actually a shy person. After my first or second tequila, however, my walls would come down, I'd stop caring so much, my insecurities would disappear, and I'd transform into a happy-go-lucky free spirit. I loved being that way, and drinking got me there.

So, I drilled down on that further.

*Why do you need to drink to have that confidence? Well, there are things I'm insecure about.*

*Okay, why are you insecure about those things? Well, because this person made me feel bad about them when I was a kid.*

Again, I just dug down deep to the root of the issue.

I wanted to become the fun, carefree version of myself without drinking. I made that my new goal: to be more like Smashton without getting smashed.

About a month after I stopped drinking, I went to New York for the *Below Deck* season seven reunion show. This gave me a chance to apologize in person to Kate for the first time since seeing the way I'd treated her. We spoke briefly off camera and some more on camera for the show. Then, after everyone discussed various big moments from the season, I also announced my new sobriety.

All of this helped me find a sense of resolution about everything that had happened and feel as though I could close the *Below Deck* chapter of my life for good. I was grateful for the experiences I'd had on the show, and now I felt grateful to move on.

# CHAPTER 24

Upon my return to St. Pete, to my surprise, some people on social media still had some problems with me announcing my sobriety the way I had. Some said I faked it for the show. Others said I hadn't stopped drinking soon enough. Those comments didn't matter to me. If anything, they just made me dive deeper and reminded me to keep myself shielded from outside noise. After all, one of the big reasons I'd had such a bad reaction in the first place came from not managing the external stimulus of my environment around me.

To that end, I treated this as ongoing practice in learning how to tune out negative distractions and not care what anybody else thought about me. This gave me good reinforcement for my new path, forcing me to focus on my reason for doing this in the first place: to become a healthier person for myself.

But, naturally, just as I started settling into a healthy sense of momentum with my personal development and sobriety, life took another one of its turns.

Around March 2020, my visa expired, requiring me to return to South Africa. While I was there, COVID-19 hit the fan. The world went into lockdown, rendering me stuck in Johannesburg again and ultimately leading to the end of my relationship with the woman in St. Pete. In a way, that proved to be a blessing in disguise, helping both of us realize that, although we'd shared a wonderful time together, we weren't quite the proper fit for a more long-term relationship. While that hurt at first, of course, I reminded myself of the implicate order of the universe and looked for the good that could come from this unexpected turn of events. Now, I had to begin focusing on my future sooner than I likely would have otherwise.

As part of that, I also felt a pull away from working on yachts. Having realized I lacked the genuine desire to become a boat captain, I felt that after *Below Deck,* yachting had little more to offer me in terms of personal development. Same as my girlfriend from St. Pete, yacht work had given me wonderful life experience and helped me grow in ways I couldn't imagine having grown otherwise. At the same time, I could see it was not meant to last my whole life. My goal was to continue to develop as a person. As I considered what an ongoing career in the industry might offer me, I no longer saw a clear sense of how yachting would help me achieve that goal. My feet needed another boat.

Instead, my mind kept turning toward a search for a career that would allow me to help people by sharing all that I had learned so far. I wanted my pain to have purpose. In parallel, I also wanted my work to be put toward building a business of my own that could grow along with me.

As maddening as the COVID lockdown was, it forced me to simply sit in my place and map out what I could do next with my life and my career. As I imagined the possibilities, I began to consider something I'd discussed with my personal trainer in Florida. My entire life, I'd loved fitness. Even in my lowest and most lonely moments, training had brought me peace, joy, and a sense of accomplishment. No matter what else might have been going wrong in my life, by taking care of my body, I maintained forward momentum for my health.

And especially now, keeping myself physically healthy helped me also improve my emotional and psychological health.

While working on *The Gene Machine,* I'd loved giving that family those personal training sessions. Likewise for when I'd worked at the yacht owner's house in Croatia, building his home gym and training him and his wife every morning. Training people made them happy and helped them stay healthy. Plus, if I did a training business the right way, it could grow over time, allowing me to help more and more people.

While sitting at home alone in South Africa, wondering how I could do that with gyms worldwide locked down, I realized that an online training business would offer me the ability to connect with clients anywhere, meaning I could make a difference for an unlimited number of people by helping them improve their overall wellness. In addition, this sort of business would provide me the flexibility to continue my pursuit of better emotional and psychological health, allowing me to continue growing as a person in the ways that felt most important to me.

After exploring various ideas of how to approach such a venture, I invested in a business coach who helped me bring my vision to life. My time working on yachts was over, but now this fitness business offered me a whole new life. One journey's end allowed another to begin.

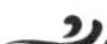

In the meantime, I began to focus again on doing deeper work to better understand and heal myself. The more I examined my relationship with alcohol, the more I realized that when I was drunk, my subconscious mind took over for my conscious mind. In recalling the lessons I'd learned about the subconscious and the power it holds, this led me to further analyze what sorts of beliefs and ideas had been drilled into me since childhood. When my subconscious took control, that's what it operated out of. Emotional tags rose to the surface, and reactions to old traumas I'd tried to bury came bursting forth.

The more I dug in and started to sense these things, strangely enough, the *worse* I felt. The more work I did on myself, the more difficult feelings came up. For a while, I thought my frustrations were with alcohol itself, and those frustrations were valid. I've seen a lot of people do a lot of drugs in my life, and I've never seen any drug bring out the absolute worst in people as consistently as alcohol does—and yet it's the easiest drug on the planet to access. While it plays an enormous role in most people's social lives, it often proves a defining factor in destroying countless people's careers, relationships, and happiness. As I spent a few months sober and continued to better calm the noise in my mind and control my external environment, I realized how much I'd been using alcohol as a stimulus to distract me from, as well as numb, my pain. I wondered how different past relationships would have played out had I not so often been under the influence of alcohol.

But my angst ran deeper than society's alcohol problem. I kept asking questions, and they kept taking me deeper, lowering my walls, showing me ways that, when I was drunk, I had allowed old, raw, emotional, painful parts of me to emerge. But beyond the vague yet obvious connection to my father and childhood, I had no clear understanding of what exactly that meant about me and how it applied to my life.

I knew I had some demons. I *felt* them, but I couldn't *see* them. And I didn't know how to understand them if they remained invisible to me.

Then, around June 2020, a cousin of mine gave me the crucial advice I needed.

# CHAPTER 25

One Friday night that summer, accompanied by my cousin's fiancé, Wesley, and my old friend Glen, I drove to a farm outside of town in an area called Magaliesburg. After spending about an hour on the highway, we turned off on a dirt road, followed for a while, and eventually approached a gate. After passing through, we continued down more dirt road until we reached the main house on the farm. From there, we kept going until we had crested a hill in the distance.

The area's landscape was beautiful—like art in nature with rivers and mountains and long, sprawling vistas. It also happened to be near the Cradle of Humankind where humanity started to exist.

Here at the top of the hill, we disembarked from the car with our things and settled into our accommodations for the weekend: small, round tents containing one bed or a bunk bed. A community kitchen and toilet were located in a corner of the campground. Just beyond the tents, a large, grassy area surrounded by some concrete steps formed a small cove. Next to that was a big, circular space under a thatched roof, and beyond that was a beautiful rock pool.

Stepping past all of this, I took in the view of an expansive, breathtaking valley. Being in this place made me feel grounded and safe, connected to the earth, and removed from everything else that normally filled my life. Out here, there was no cell phone service, internet, or television. Just us, the earth, and each other. And the medicine. Looking over this valley and taking in my surroundings, I felt a clear sense of exactly why I was here and the work I was here to do.

About a half-dozen other people soon joined me, Glen, and Wesley, and we gathered in the cove with a kind, warm woman named Michelle. After going through introductions, Michelle asked us to consider our goals for the weekend—why we were there.

We were here to partake in what my cousin had described to me as "plant medicine." Having attended one such ceremony with Wesley recently, she'd told me this helped them better understand themselves—especially their subconscious minds—and changed their lives.

After journeying to this farm, they spent a couple of days undergoing a "plant medicine ceremony." The ceremony involved drinking teas brewed from plants that would generate psychedelic experiences and hallucinations, which would ultimately bring buried and formative parts of their subconscious to the surface. This lasted for hours, throughout an entire night, and usually came with vomiting and diarrhea. Essentially, the ceremony provided a purge in every sense, from the physical to the mental and emotional to the spiritual.

Over the course of the weekend, the ceremony would begin with one night of drinking an intense brew from the *Banisteriopsis caapi* vine commonly known as Ayahuasca, followed by a day of drinking a milder tea called San Pedro brewed from cacti. I'd never heard of San Pedro, and I'd only heard of Ayahuasca once when an old college friend had told me about the time he'd tried it and hated it. Saying the experience was one of the worst in his entire life, he told me about seeing demons and visiting hell. Far from a glowing recommendation.

Nevertheless, my cousin thought this could provide me with one of the most healing experiences I had ever encountered. The medicine brings up memories, often ones that have been repressed but which correlate with pain you've been carrying your entire life. It's meant to help you understand parts of yourself that you may not have otherwise had access to, preventing you from being able to heal from things you may never have known or had forgotten.

I've since learned that the psychedelic compounds active in Ayahuasca and San Pedro are being isolated and studied by various scientists as clinical means by which to treat various mental illnesses and traumas. Somehow, ancient shamans discovered the formulas for brewing these teas and passed down that knowledge from generation to generation until it survived here in our modern world.

I thought this sounded phenomenal, and I was eager to try it. This seemed like the perfect next adventure. My cousin gave me fair warning, however, that the experience would be intense, challenge me like I'd never been challenged before, and, in her words, "put me on my ass."

I said let's do it, so my cousin put me in touch with Michelle to make the arrangements. Leading up to the ceremony, Michelle told me to go on a strict diet, cutting out processed foods, sugar, and anything except the simplest, cleanest foods in order to give my body and mind a clear system for receiving the medicine.

Now, here I was with Michelle beginning to guide us through the process as we sat in the large circular outdoor area under the thatched shelter. After making sure we all felt familiar with our surroundings and each other, Michelle guided us to set our intentions for the journey that the medicine would take us on and reminded us to remain open to whatever form that journey took. Ultimately, she said, the medicine would take us where we needed to go.

I wanted to keep my first experience with the medicine light and exploratory, possessing no deep desire to meet any demons or visit hell. With my business going well, and recognizing that, with this business, I could live and work anywhere in the world, I hoped to gain insights into how to better run my company. Plus, I hoped to develop a clearer sense of direction for where I should be going next in my life.

Then, it was time to take our first dose of Ayahuasca.

After drinking from a cup containing a small serving of earthy liquid, I sat on a mat with my eyes closed and a bucket for my vomit beside me, waiting for the effects to take hold. People around me began to breathe hard and writhe and groan as the Ayahuasca took them, and others started to weep. Meanwhile, after quite some time had passed, I felt nothing. Michelle gave me a second dose and then a third. Everyone around me was falling deep into what seemed to be an incredibly profound experience. Meanwhile, I sat there motionless, trying to keep my eyes closed, experiencing nothing.

"How are you feeling?" Michelle asked me.

"I'm not really feeling anything," I said.

"Interesting," she replied thoughtfully.

She looked over at Wesley sitting across the room from me and told me that he was having the same non-experience. "There's a deeper connection between you two," she said. "You should see if you can find it."

As she spoke, and as my mind processed her words, her voice suddenly dropped several octaves, and she sounded like she was speaking incredibly slowly. Her face began to contort and move in a wavy fashion, and all my other senses began to intensify and slow down all at once, almost as though I had gone for a dive into the sea.

As she finished speaking, I suddenly recalled a conversation I'd had with Wesley before. In a distant corner of my mind, I heard Wesley's voice discussing his father and some of the painful issues they had between them. Then, I thought of my own father. I began to feel some things with clarity and certainty the way you acutely feel water when you walk into the ocean.

That was our connection. We both carried pain from our fathers.

Michelle's voice faded, and her face blurred, and the same happened with everything else around me, my consciousness slipping into the deep of an oncoming psychological onslaught. The medicine had begun its work on me.

Throughout the evening, I experienced massive waves of intense emotion and memory, my entire life moving through my mind as though something were carrying me through my past. I relived myriad interactions and conversations and incidents, particularly those from my youngest years. Some of these were fun, others were argumentative, and yet others were sad. When I questioned why the medicine was taking me here, I sensed that this was to prepare me for something else to come, as though I needed these memories to prime me for deeper and more intense memories.

Eventually, I reached a point of exhaustion where I craved sleep but couldn't actually fall into slumber. Then, I began to vomit, a reaction that lasted for quite some time. When I finished with that, I finally slept.

After we awoke the next day, we drank a bit of water but ate nothing before initiating another ceremony, this time with San Pedro, a much gentler medicine. The Ayahuasca shook things up; the San Pedro helped us process what Ayahuasca had shown us. After receiving our portion of San Pedro, we were encouraged to find a quiet area of our own, enjoy the beautiful scenery, and trust the medicine to do its work with us. I spent a wonderful morning experiencing warmth and safety, as though the medicine were offering me comfort after a challenging night full of rough emotion and purging. However, I also still sensed that I was being prepared for something even more challenging to come.

That afternoon, we gathered together to share some fruit in a small breaking of our fast. As I ate some grapes, strawberries, and papaya, I thought they were the best-tasting fruit I'd ever had in my entire life.

Michelle turned on some music and encouraged us to dance as we prepared for the next phase of the ceremony. She told us to simply move in whatever way we felt led, allowing our bodies to help us explore and process and integrate all we had felt and experienced so far. I found myself doing these slow, rhythmic movements akin to yoga poses, feeling the desire to stretch and sweat with a vague sense that I needed to further prepare myself for . . . something.

As we danced, one of the men in the group began to cry in deep, mournful howls, and I found myself pulled toward him as he curled into a ball on the ground. I placed my hands on the earth beside him, wanting him to feel safe and know that everything was going to be okay. While providing him with that comfort, suddenly, I wasn't in Magaliesburg anymore but rather in my childhood bedroom with my little brother, doing the same thing for him as he cried while our father screamed and broke things outside our door.

In a flash, I was re-experiencing parts of my childhood when this sort of thing happened regularly with me offering solace to my baby brother while he cried in confusion and fear. He was so young. I relived a number of moments like that, and I relived the way I grew up feeling a continual need to protect my brother from the anger and chaos that often surrounded us.

As I again experienced this period of my youth, I reconnected with an emotion I constantly shoved aside at the time: I *also* felt intense confusion and fear, and sometimes, I felt like my heart was breaking, too, same as my baby brother's. As he cried, I wanted to cry; as I held him, I wanted to be held. But I couldn't because I felt like someone in our family needed to be strong and keep their shit together, so I hardened myself against any feelings that threatened my sense of strength.

This was the first challenge that made me feel overwhelmed, that I then learned to face down and overcome, and I did it over and over and over again. I lived my life refusing to allow those emotions to exist, refusing to feel that fear, refusing to believe just how difficult of a situation this was, needing to be strong and secure so that my brother felt safe with somebody.

Then, I returned to the present, to the ceremony in Magaliesburg, where I *was* safe, and I broke down. I cried for hours, a soreness filling my heart like water entering through a hole in the bottom of a boat. An ache suffused my chest, and the more I cried, the deeper that ache became. Before long, Michelle came to sit with me without saying a word, and her mere presence made me feel safe and loved and held. I tried to tell her what I was experiencing, but I could hardly speak, only able to say two words on repeat: "It hurts."

For four hours, I just sat there and remembered and felt things that I'd ignored all my life. I just kept crying, feeling completely out of control. Michelle stayed with me, giving me the support and care I'd needed all those years. After so much time carrying all of this on my own, now I had someone here with me, giving me the comfort I'd always given someone else and longed for myself.

The only other words I could find were these: "I've got to let it go. I've got to let it go."

"Yes," Michelle said. "And you can. You can."

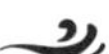

Later that afternoon, with twilight on the horizon, the ceremony came to an end. After composing myself, I joined the circle in the cove with everyone else. We were supposed to share from our experiences, and everyone else seemed to have finished their process and gained a clear understanding of what the medicine had taught them this weekend. I did not share their sense of closure or understanding. When it was my turn, I struggled to find any words that could suffice, and I still felt full of emotion that didn't seem like it would abate any time soon. As I tried to speak, I broke down in tears once again.

The weekend was coming to an end, and everyone else seemed to have embarked on, and then returned from, healing journeys of cosmic proportions. But I still felt like I was somewhere else, not having returned from my journey yet. During my ceremony, the more I'd said, "I've got to let it go," the more I *felt it,* and the less I felt like I was actually letting anything go.

While everyone stayed up talking and eating some vegetable soup, I went to bed, needing space and time for myself, hoping to further process my experience. I tried to sleep, but couldn't, and then, I began to cry again.

Quite abruptly, my mind took me somewhere else. This time, I saw flashes of myself submerged in a body of water, trying to look up and see out of it and feeling intense animosity and rage. I felt trapped, or caught, as though someone were holding me underwater. Through the haze, I saw the face of my mother's uncle—my grandmother's brother—and I felt a deeply confusing but intensely real sense of anger toward him. I was furious at him for trying to hurt me.

When the moment faded, I stopped crying and went to the ceremony leader. "I think," I said, "somebody tried to kill me when I was young."

Finally, I found the words to express all I had experienced, and we had a long conversation. Michelle told me that this had been a good experience for me, but this was only the beginning. The medicine had shown me some deep truths about myself, but I still needed to find healthy means by which to process them and integrate them into my life. As we talked, I realized that my next task was to go to my mother or father and ask them what they might know about this newly rediscovered memory.

Then, I ate. I rejoined the group and, starving, devoured a big bowl of vegetable soup. Waves of emotion continued to wash over me, and calm tears kept leaking out of my eyes as I felt deep love and appreciation for this moment and all that it was giving me.

# CHAPTER 26

About a week later, I met my father for lunch at The Salsa Grill, a Mexican restaurant where we often ate together. On this day, the place was quiet and full of empty tables, and the environment felt comfortable for a heavy conversation.

After a bit of small talk, I told him about the plant medicine ceremony. Feeling only curiosity and love and wanting him to feel the same, I chose my words and my tone carefully as I told him about the process of experiencing old and forgotten memories and emotions. This led into my memory of being in a body of water where I felt like somebody was trying to kill me when I was very young.

By the way he shifted in his chair and the expression that took shape on his face, I could tell he was in a bit of shock at what I was saying.

Gently, I asked him if he happened to know anything about that.

"You really remember that?" he said. "Has it really affected you?"

"Sort of," I said. "I'm just not really sure *what* actually happened."

With no additional prompting, he told me the story.

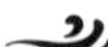

After my mom discovered that she was pregnant at sixteen years old, her father and brother—my grandfather and "uncle"—had been vehemently opposed to her going through with the pregnancy and urged her to get an abortion. My mom's family carried a great deal of concern for maintaining a certain image and reputation, and their daughter becoming pregnant at such a young age did not fit in with that.

When my mother felt uncertain about having the abortion, they became quite insistent about the matter—with my uncle serving as the primary aggressor. As my mom deliberated and continued to express doubt, my uncle rallied the men in her family together with a plan to physically force her to go to the abortion clinic.

Upon hearing about this plan, my dad, at seventeen years old, drove to her house and arrived just as all the men did, at which point he proceeded to engage them in a series of aggressive encounters. Then, he took my mom to go live with him and his mother, where he would keep her and their baby safe.

Where he would keep me safe.

As I listened to his story, I felt peace take hold inside of me. This felt true, and this explained so much. That memory I had, of being underwater, of my uncle trying to kill me, had all taken place when I was still the size of a pea in my mother's womb.

And my dad . . . My dad had literally fought my mother's family off to keep them from forcing her to have an abortion—to have *me* aborted.

My dad had fought for me to be born.

I'd had no idea the extent to which he had put his neck on the line for me and my mom back then. Likewise, I'd never been fully aware of how deep the tension ran between my dad and my mom's family. But now I knew.

Overcome with heartfelt appreciation for what he'd done to bring me into the world and raise me, I thanked him. When I said that, he softened in a way I'd never quite seen before, and he smiled, a new lightness and joy entering his eyes. We shared a big, emotional hug, both of us shaking a bit from the intensity of it all. The beauty of the moment hung thick in the air for me, as I felt like we were two people who'd known each other forever and yet, somehow, had only just met. I felt like I truly understood my dad for the first time in my life.

After that lunch, we continued to talk more often, and he gradually opened up to me. The more I learned about him, the more empathy I felt for him. Out of respect for others involved, I feel the need to keep the details of these conversations private, but I came to see that, clearly, my dad had endured some deep and challenging issues in his relationships with my mom and, later, my brother's mom. He was a man who loved fiercely and passionately, and he didn't always receive that same love in return.

The more I learned about his life and relationships, the more I came to understand what the plant medicine ceremony had been trying to teach me about my relationship with him: *Let it go.* Yes, the anger that would come exploding out of me sometimes—that *was* related to my dad's behavior as I was growing up. But my big epiphany, the big answer for me here, wasn't about pushing him away or cutting him out of my life or forgetting all about him. My epiphany was this: *It's not about me.* My big answer was to entrench myself in understanding in order to deepen my empathy for him.

As I did so, my entire perspective on him underwent a dynamic shift, and I saw how his life and emotional history had had such a direct effect on me—the ways they intertwined.

And yet, at the same time, I no longer needed to hold onto that. Now that I understood him, I felt as though I understood myself. My anger had just come from pain. The same was true for him. And now that I knew how to forgive him, I could also forgive myself.

I felt the same as when the tender line had been released from the yacht right when I thought I was going to watch my foot get ripped off.

I felt peace.

# EPILOGUE

As I work on this book right now, it is two and a half years later in the winter of 2022. I'm still sober, and I'm sitting in a townhome in Raleigh, North Carolina, in the United States, where I am living with the love of my life, Sarah. The implicate order of the universe has certainly kept my life interesting with unexpected twists and turns, and she is by far the most unexpected and interesting—and welcome—of them all. My love story with her is the epitome of finding security in the unknown, and how things have developed with her encapsulates everything I've learned along this crazy journey. If I'd never learned all that I did—if I'd never let myself be torn apart—I doubt I could have found the love I have with her.

Things with Sarah began, in a way, all the way back in January 2020 when I was living in Johannesburg with Glen during lockdown. Sarah was living in London, where she was ending a marriage of eight years and moving in with some of her friends. Those friends, Adam and Roxy, just so happened to also be friends of mine from school. They joked with her about setting us up, saying that she reminded them of a female version of me, but. Of course, our lives were far too separate for anything like that to happen just yet. That was likely for the best, as I still had a lot of growing to do at that point. Roxy and

Adam had some concerns that, in all of my Smashtonian party boy glory at the time, I might not be the best fit for dear, sweet Sarah.

Later, I called Adam and Roxy to congratulate them on their pregnancy. Unbeknownst to me, in the background of that call, Roxy had told Sarah I was on the phone, so the two of them eavesdropped on my conversation with Adam until he got annoyed and fled to a bedroom. After he and I talked for half an hour and he emerged again, Sarah waited with bated breath, wondering what all Adam had told me about her.

Adam hadn't told me a thing.

A few months later, Sarah decided to move back to her hometown in Michigan for a little while, needing to reconnect with friends and family there for the sake of her mental health as she navigated the turbulence of life post-divorce. She remembered Adam mentioning that I had mentioned to *him* that I was planning to return to the States after South Africa. So, feeling as though she had nothing to lose, Sarah threw caution to the wind and fired off a direct message to me on Instagram. Why Instagram, you might ask? Adam had refused to give her my number, telling her that she was too good for me.

Well, Sarah introduced herself, we got to chatting, and we never really stopped. I was fresh off of dating someone else, trying to get a new business off the ground, and living a life that felt completely unpredictable. She was going through a divorce. Neither of us had relationships on the brain, making things feel relaxed and just friendly between us. There was something wonderful about that.

We each had somebody new in our lives who felt completely separate from our lives at the same time. No topic felt off limits, and neither of us ever felt judged by the other. With no history together but enough friends in common to have a level of mutual comfort with no preconceived notions or pressure, we met each other right where we were.

We'd each check in once a day or so to see how the other was doing. With every conversation, we'd listen to each other vent, tell each other stories about our lives, and simply offer each other the support we needed when we needed it. In hindsight, we were giving one another far more support than we realized at the time—and that's beautiful. Clearly, we needed each other more than we thought.

Inevitably, our bond deepened, emotions became more involved, and the situation began to feel a bit serious. Naturally, that freaked me out. To that point, remember, all my life had felt chaotic and stressful. That's all I knew. Of course, that also extended to my various romantic relationships. In fact, that likely *most* affected my romantic relationships. When you begin to fall in love with somebody, that opens you up to parts of yourself perhaps most sensitive to past pain and trauma. After all that I had been through, getting too close to anyone absolutely terrified me. So, not only was I learning how to trust Sarah, but I was also still learning how to trust myself.

I had a conversation with her that, in my mind, meant the end of things between us. I gave her some speech about how much I liked her but indicated I wasn't ready for the commitment of being in a full relationship. I stated that this was starting to feel that way, but I needed to be focusing more on my business and getting my life together. After ending the call, I felt terrible and sad, but she had received things with tremendous grace and compassion and understanding, for which I also felt grateful.

Well, she called me again the very next day and then the day after that and so on. She just kept checking in on me, being there for me, and offering her support. The truth was, I *needed* that support.

With the benefit of hindsight, I later realized that when I had tried to end things with her, one of my biggest fears had been that I would hurt her due to my commitment issues. She had become a special person in my life, an invaluable friend with a beautiful heart, someone who meant a great deal to me. I wanted to take care of her heart, and I was concerned that I wasn't equipped to do so at that time. She later made the point that this actually showed a lot of growth and maturity on my part because a more selfish person would have simply used her for her support until they had gotten all that they needed out of her.

My other biggest fear was that I was becoming a burden to her, and I felt that by creating distance between us, I would spare her from being weighed down by all my shit. Bear in mind, much of this began to unfold as we lived thousands of miles apart from each other, in separate countries on separate continents, while I was going through the darkest time of my life in the wake of what I'd seen in myself on that last season of *Below Deck.*

Nevertheless, Sarah saw everything I was dealing with, and she continued caring for me anyway, not only with her words but with her actions. She became a steady, calm, consistent presence in my life the likes of which I had rarely known. All of that even after I had tried to push her away.

She really was like the female version of me. As you've seen throughout this book, I've always been the person who decides what he wants and refuses to give up on trying to get it. Looking back, we realized that Sarah was doing that with me. She just said to herself, *Well, I really like this guy, and I want to keep being there for him.* So, she did in her calm, sweet, thoughtful little ways. Often, that was as simple as giving me a call. And, of course, I didn't *really* want to be done with her because I kept answering when her name flashed across my phone screen.

I found myself feeling immense appreciation and respect for that, and at some point, I said the same thing she did. *I really like this girl.*

On a deeper psychological level, I was able to accept how much I liked her because I'd begun to like myself more as a person—which enabled me to more deeply accept that someone *I* liked could *also* really like *me.*

I could tell her anything, even stories about myself that I thought made me look crazy or stupid or like a bad person. Instead of making me feel judged, she typically had a way of making me like myself more for the things I had done. She would laugh, offer advice, and provide a perspective I'd never thought of that struck me as profound and insightful and true. She made me feel seen. And not only did she really see me, but instead of that making her disappear, like I feared it would, it only cemented our bond. I needed someone like her more than I knew until I was experiencing it—I needed someone who liked me simply for who I was, not who they thought I should be.

As much healing as we can do single and alone, and as necessary as times of solitude can be, nothing offers the level of healing that a kind and loving relationship can provide.

One of the most healing parts of all was the way she felt that I was doing the same for her. Where I was learning not to run from love, she was learning not to hold onto love too tight. Later, she told me that I had this way of recognizing tendencies in her that exhibited that urge to grasp too hard and helped her ease her grip—all without making her feel bad for being that way. I just reminded her that she didn't need to do such things because now, although neither of us could predict the future, I wasn't going to run from her. I wasn't going anywhere.

We both learned to stop putting expectations on things. Employing some of the lessons I'd learned, we worked to retrain our subconscious so that our past experiences didn't have a negative influence on our present reality. We taught ourselves to believe in the good that existed now. In accepting what we had for what it was, we let ourselves simply enjoy it all.

Just as I'd been shamed by people for what I perceived as my flaws, she had as well. But just as she never thought any of my flaws made me broken or bad, I believed the same thing about her. We were just two people learning how to live—and how to love.

For months, all of this happened over the phone, one video chat after another from thousands of miles apart.

After a few months with her family in Michigan, Sarah accepted a job in Raleigh. I met her there. By this point, I'd begun to focus on my fitness business, giving me the flexibility to go where I wanted pretty much whenever I wanted. And I wanted to be with her.

She picked me up from the airport, and for our first date, we went to a restaurant called Rosewater near her apartment in Raleigh's North

Hills neighborhood. Our plan had been for me to stay in the Raleigh area for one week, maybe two.

Instead, I stayed six months.

Once we saw each other in person, we were so excited to finally be together that we fell into total and complete infatuation. All we had in her apartment was a chair and bed, without even a table or anything else for a long time, and that was all we needed. She'd go to work, and I would work in the kitchen at the counter. When she'd come home after her workday, we would make dinner together and talk.

We didn't watch much TV. On the occasions we did leave the apartment, we would play tennis, go to the gym, and take long walks and hikes around the Raleigh area, one of the most unique places I have ever lived. Although it has the population, amenities, and entertainment of a big city, the area has more suburban and rural vibes with endless hills, a massive number of pines and oaks and other trees, and beautiful trails through countless vibrant forests, which feel wonderful to get lost in.

Despite me technically moving in on our first date, Sarah and I took care to avoid putting too many expectations on our situation, but by this point, we had spent so much time talking that we realized we had already built a nice, clean, strong foundation for ourselves. I overthought things for a little while at first, knowing that my job allowed me to go anywhere I wanted, which was perfect for someone with all the commitment issues that I had. I worried at times whether being here with her in Raleigh was right for me and whether this would take me the right direction for my life. And I worried that I wasn't ready for all of this.

However, the more time I spent with her, the more I realized how much I loved being with her, and my energy began to turn away from those worries and focus more on taking care of what we had. I had a great boat here, so I got in with both feet.

You'll remember from throughout the book that when things start to go well for me, I have to get ready for something bad to happen. The good thing now was that I was able to recognize that and avoid acting on my self-destructive impulses. Instead, I confided in Sarah. She reassured me that she wasn't going anywhere. She wasn't going to do anything to jeopardize our relationship. She loved me, and she was going to do her part to take care of us. Likewise, she said that she also always found herself waiting for the other shoe to drop, so to speak. Even now, she says some part of her is just waiting for things to go bad somehow.

So, we talk about it. We discuss the thoughts we are having. We do this as we've done everything else together: with no judgment, with no ego, without one of us making our negative thoughts the other person's fault. It is as though we both know how to just let each other be . . . human.

We reassure each other. We realize we've both felt the same way. And that's hilarious, once we talk through it because the reason we both feel this way is, really, we both just feel so grateful that we found each other—almost like we can't believe it. In this big, crazy world, after all the things I have done, after all that Sarah has been through, for both of us to somehow know Adam and Roxy, to be introduced to each other through them, and for that to lead to this—we just feel so damn lucky. Naturally, sometimes, that also makes us feel a lot of fear that somehow, someday, that luck will run out, and all of this will go away. But we have faith in our future and in each other.

Of course, we have our struggles. We both get freaked out by the commitment of it all. We're aware that we have work to do. But that work is done in a loving way. For her, she's never been in a relationship with someone who, in her words, "actually speaks to me" and "is actually fun." She's always been considered a serious person by her family and siblings, but to me, she's not only this smart, warm, caring woman—she's also this big goofball. Apparently, I bring it out in her. And that's funny to me because my goofy side comes out with her so much more simply because she's so good at making me feel comfortable just being who I am. That's what we both want. She likes to say that one day we're going to be old and gray, and when those days come, we're just going to want somebody we can talk to.

The great thing about the way our friendship began, too, is that all we had for the first ten months or so was phone calls and video chat. We learned so many nuances about each other's moods and communication styles and tones that, now, we can immediately tell when one of us is feeling off just by the way we say a word. And we know how to talk through it because all we did for almost a year was talk.

We laugh and joke around and be silly all the time too. It's not all serious conversations about all the terrible shit in our lives—the traumas we've been through and are healing from. In a lot of ways, I think the most healing thing you can do is stop focusing on your healing and just live your life with as much joy as you can find. But to do that, you have to be at peace with yourself, and I've never been with someone who made me feel 100 percent comfortable being 100 percent myself the way that she does.

The way that she loves me, the way that she supports me, and simply the way that she is as a human being makes me feel like what we have is enough. Anything else we might want we can find in each other and in this relationship. Of course, all relationships take work—but good relationships hold space for that work to be done in harmony together.

As I realized this, my perception continued to evolve. I improved in my ability to separate my present from my past and see how to create my own future. I can be happy with this woman. I can be happy with my life. I can break the cycle of loss. I can have what I want and let it be good. I can be in a relationship with somebody I love and who I can trust to love me. I can be in a relationship and not worry about enduring the same struggles that my parents had. I can be in love, and have somebody be in love with me, and still be at peace.

At some point with Sarah, I realized with blinding clarity how that had been my core issue. Relationships, both with others and with myself, had always been the tender line wrapped around my ankle, pulling me apart. In that metaphor, the yacht was where the relationship could go, a place of love and joy that could carry me into a beautiful life; the tender was all the pain and heartache and conflict that I saw destroy one relationship after another, which became engrained in me as inevitable.

All my life, I'd let the tender tear me in two over and over again. I'd find myself in pain as I drove this little boat behind the big, beautiful yacht where I could see other people all happy and serene, never knowing how to join them there. Now, with Sarah, we were on a big, beautiful yacht of our own making.

One day this past summer, Sarah drove me to the Raleigh airport, tearful and sad. I was leaving. Having been in and out of the States over the course of two years, taking care of various business and visa matters, I had to make another trip to Portugal and, from there, to South Africa. Depending on how long some things took, months might pass before I could return. I had been planning the trip for weeks, and the build-up to this departure seemed to fill me with dread. We had grown so close to each other that leaving again just felt harder than ever for both of us. It just didn't feel right for us to be apart.

Emotions ran high as we arrived, and I asked her to come into the airport with me, saying I wanted as much time with her as I could get before I had to go through security. We parked, I gathered my things, and we walked through the parking deck and down to the terminal, a backpack slung over my shoulders and a rolling carry-on bag in my hand. As we made our way through the airport doors and approached security, I suggested taking a selfie at the place she and I had first met in person when Sarah had picked me up from the airport.

Once again, life seemed to be pulling me in two different directions, and she told me she wished I didn't have to go. I told her, "There is only one way that I do not get on that plane right now, and that's if you answer the next question correctly."

She looked at me in complete confusion and shock. "*What?* What do you mean . . . You're not leaving?"

I lowered myself down to one knee, reached in my pocket, pulled out a ring, and asked her, "Will you marry me? In response, she lowered herself down to my level and completely broke down in my arms. I knew how badly she wanted this of us, and I did not want to live another day without her . . . She said yes!

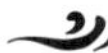

Now, after all the work I had done on myself, and after the love Sarah had shown me, I'd learned how to let the tender line go. To stop stepping into it and letting it rip me off the yacht.

Yachts need a tender, and life and love and relationships all come with their own pain. But the key is learning to let the pain be useful—to take you to new places you never thought you could go. That's how you become the person you always wanted to be and live a life you always wanted live.

I hope sharing my story like this has helped you with your own story. I still have a lot of work to do, but now, I'm grateful for the hard times I've endured, the lessons I've learned, and the ways I've grown. I still don't always know exactly where life is going, but at least now, I feel like I know how to live.